Trauma *to*
TRIUMPH

A PATH TO WHOLENESS, HAPPINESS AND PERSONAL POWER THROUGH AWARENESS

Trauma *to* TRIUMPH

A PATH TO WHOLENESS, HAPPINESS AND PERSONAL POWER THROUGH AWARENESS

D. LYNN ANDERSON

Published by Best Seller Publishing®, St. Augustine, FL
Best Seller Publishing® is a registered trademark.
Printed in the United States of America.
ISBN: 978-1-956649-82-6

For more information, please write:
Best Seller Publishing®
53 Marine Street
St. Augustine, FL 32084
or call 1 (626) 765-9750
Visit us online at: www.BestSellerPublishing.org

TABLE OF CONTENTS

DEDICATION

To Siobhán and Cillian, my greatest teachers

SPECIAL THANKS

I am deeply grateful to those who helped keep me sane and focused during the writing of this book. I am indebted to Karl, Lala & Uncle, Shantelle, Valerie, Janice, as well as a handful of friends, family, mentors and classmates. Also, Matt S., Anna R., Adrien B. and Rob K. at Best Seller Publishing were indispensable. This book would not have been possible without the help of all of them.

FOREWORD

You hold in your hands a book that is a wonderful guide to lead you down a path of clarity, healing and freedom so that you can reclaim the life that you are meant to live.

Whether you are aware of trauma from your past or you cannot identify anything in particular but have a sense that there is something from your past that is constricting or inhibiting your freedom to live and express the truth of who you are fully, this book is a lovely guide to give you the clarity and the tools that can assist you to move forward to create a more fulfilling and joyful life for yourself.

Lynn has walked her talk. She shares in this book her own journey of emotional neglect and childhood trauma, and how her knowledge of this remained buried for years, negatively impacting her relationships and how she lived her life. She boldly shares with you what led to her awakening to the truth of her trauma, and her healing journey that followed, leading to her living the triumphant life she now enjoys, while also helping others to heal and transcend their emotional trauma.

In these pages are various processes for you to put into action right away, so that you can dive deep into your own layers, gain more clarity and practically apply exercises that will support you.

As you read through these pages, I encourage you to feel into how Lynn's story relates to your own life. Take the time to go through all the exercises she provides for you and apply them. I

believe that as you do this, you can start creating a shift and step
into the next chapter of your life, one that is more fulfilling, authentic, peaceful and expressed. Use this book to give more clarity and
insight into your own journey, transcend your emotional wounds
and turn trauma into your triumph.

—Jaitara Jayde, author of
The Four Sacred Laws of Sexual Enlightenment,
facilitator of feminine empowerment and intimacy coach

INTRODUCTION

As far as stories go, mine probably appears pretty run-of-the-mill from most people's perspective. I grew up middle-class in the '70s, in the suburbs with my parents, my older sister and the family dog (there were four over the years). We lived in a sleepy neighborhood, because in my town, many of them were back then. I spent my days doing homework and hanging out with my friends from school, often staying late after class. Even after my friends had long since gone, I stayed in order to avoid going home, where chores and ennui awaited. Fast-forward a few years to when I met my high school sweetheart, whom I'll call Mark (who would later become my husband). I went to a prestigious art college after high school, and I started making independent films with Mark and our friends in our free time. We even moved to Los Angeles for a short period, to work on independent films and student productions, with ambitions of going to film school ourselves. We decided to change course, however, and ended up moving back home, getting "real" jobs and buying a house. We did a decent amount of traveling, and we renovated the house in the following decade or so.

We later decided upon having two children, which I had honestly never been keen to do before, and I had communicated this early on. In fact, I had never wanted children at all, for reasons that I did not understand at the time. However, after a lot of consideration (and some pressure from Mark), I finally bought into the idea and we took the plunge. I had a daughter in 2012 and a son in 2014, who are both wonderful, challenging and loving little goofballs ... ahem, I mean people!

It probably looks like a pretty good life by most people's estimates. I thought so too. Nothing looked amiss, even to me. I was definitely aware of my good fortune, and I was very grateful, but there was a constant gnawing at the back of my mind and an uneasiness deep in my core that grew with time. It didn't declare itself openly, but crept, quietly and insidiously, into my mind, body and soul.

I had a good life, blessed in many ways, but it never felt like *mine*. It felt like I was following some unknown script authored by someone or something else. This unacknowledged angst had affected me, without my knowing it, by coloring my every experience, my every perception, and influencing every decision I made. My marriage was a shield blocking me from the recognition of an unconscious dread hidden away inside me. It distracted me from allowing the thought—and recognizing the feeling—that I had felt for as long as I could remember: that I didn't belong.

This malaise began quietly in my childhood, but it developed into full-blown major depression by my twenties. It was my constant companion. I often slept for days, trying to escape the despair. At Mark's suggestion, I finally sought help and was prescribed some antidepressants. I used them faithfully and discovered what it felt like to feel "normal" for the first time in my life, or what I perceived to be normal, anyhow. I had a new sense of ease that had not been present before. At this point, in my thirties, I was doing better than ever before, and this is when we bought our house and traveled some.

Things were going well for a time. Once we decided to have children, I went off the antidepressants so as not to adversely affect our babies in utero. This choice would end up leading to my unraveling. That one decision set the stage to blow up almost everything in my life: first my marriage, and then a series of events that would have a chain reaction in my life, like setting off a series of depth charges under the surface of my psyche. It also ultimately led to me pursuing an education in counseling psychology and to the writing of this book. I had a lot to learn about myself in the interim, though.

For the longest time, I had no explanation for the source of my depression. I thought that it was simply my lot in life. It took years of wondering, questioning and agonizing to even realize that I was unhappy. Then I began to question why. The answer was that I wasn't leading my own life but living one that was prescribed to me by society, and that I believed others expected of me. I had spent my childhood and youth *unconsciously* doing what I believed others wanted of me, at the expense of my own soul. I was a pleaser, caught in the self-defeating loop of survival mode from childhood, and therefore I had bypassed any chance of fulfillment. I was stuck, never growing, never trusting, least of all in myself, and never knowing there was any other way to live.

Awareness about what was wrong began to creep in, persisting as my current circumstances became untenable. This led me to make irrevocable, life-altering decisions that affected my whole family. Eventually, with time and experience, I gained some insight that guided me to a comprehensive understanding of myself and what was so terribly wrong.

It started when I recognized that I wasn't happy in my marriage and tried to figure out why. I was early in the discovery process when my intuition had already vaguely tipped me off that my upbringing had something to do with why I stayed in an unhappy marriage, but I didn't make the direct connection until later. I had to drill down to find out where these ideas came from. I was just beginning to integrate the idea of childhood emotional neglect into my psyche, and to recognize everything that had led up to this point, when I had an experience that nearly destroyed me.

Less than a year after the inevitable separation from my husband, someone new had entered my life, and over the next two years he turned my emotional world upside down. The love I felt for this person—let's call him Myles—was like nothing I'd ever experienced before. To me, he was The One. After a roller coaster of emotion, difficulties with expression and communication, as well as triggering on both our parts, circumstances (and trauma) dictated that he would eventually reject me, resulting in an overwhelmingly destructive overreaction on my part. My life descended into a hellish nightmare. I had to rebuild it as a matter of survival.

Picking up the pieces of my shattered life took over eighteen months, in which time I figured out what had happened to set me up for such incredible pain, chaos and distress. I traced everything back to a childhood entirely devoid of appropriate care and attention, by both of my parents. I now know that I was loved, but I had no practical way of knowing it or feeling it as a child, because expressions of love were absent in my home, and my parents' caring for anything beyond our physical needs was inconsistent at best. This resulted in a profound lack of self-worth and self-love that dogged me throughout life. The effects of virtually no physical contact or even much attention being paid to me had embedded itself in my nervous system, manifesting in shyness and socially awkward behavior, and later social withdrawal. It was dormant for decades, thwarting emotional intimacy despite my being married at the time. Then, much later, Myles entered my life to activate my traumatic response over and over again because of the push/pull, hot/cold nature of our interactions, reenacting the trauma implanted in my youth, of trying to please someone for attention.

That traumatic response set off a cascading series of negative consequences in my life that took me those eighteen-plus months to reconcile, put back in order and heal. I had to "unpack my baggage," so to speak, to figure out why this had happened and how to get past it.

Throughout this book, I will highlight the trickle-down effect trauma had on all the areas of my rather sheltered life. I will get into the specifics of the fallout in Chapter 1. From there, I will guide you toward awareness and how to avoid any pitfalls you may encounter, instead of making a giant leap into the abyss, like me.

TRAUMA CLUES

If any part of my story sounds familiar to you, or if elements of it remind you of similar situations you have been in or feelings you may have had, you may have experienced childhood trauma, particularly in the form of emotional neglect. Other feelings can offer you clues as well. If you have ever felt that something is very wrong but you can't put your finger on it, or if you have an idea that your family upbringing has had a long-lasting negative impact on you but you don't know why, this may indicate childhood emotional neglect. If you feel desperate to change your life, you may have chronic unmet needs from your childhood, which can bleed into adulthood.

Some other signs to look for are whether you have lived feeling as though you have never been able to "speak your truth" and live according to your own values, or perhaps even give your opinion. Fundamentally, if you have never actually figured out who you are or determined your own identity, you probably have never developed a sense of self, leaving you rudderless and vulnerable to codependency or "relationship addiction." If you are waiting for "permission" to pursue your own ambitions, or even leave either your parents or your partner, this is another indication, as this was my most impactful and enduring symptom.

There are more obvious clues as well. Do you experience any of the following?

- Have difficulty entering or maintaining relationships?
- Find it hard to enter conversations and to connect with people?
- Have trouble making decisions?

- Have trouble asking for help, or even knowing when you need help?
- Feel behind, compared to others, like you are always playing catch-up?
- Feel like you are on the outside of life, looking in?
- Self-sabotage your efforts to get what you want out of life?
- Avoid conflict and have trouble standing up for yourself?
- Judge yourself more harshly than others?
- Feel empty inside and that you don't belong?

All of this can leave you feeling like no one gets you and that you are alone in your experience because you are used to having to figure it all out on your own. Perhaps you don't feel you can rely on anyone because in your childhood, no one was there for you. I answered yes to all of the above situations. Much of this can point toward emotional neglect (Webb, 2012).

TAKING A NEW PATH

If you know no alternative to how you are living your life right now, this book will show you a path to identify your trauma and create a difference in your life. If you find yourself putting your own needs last to please others and feel like it's never "your turn" to get what you want, or that you're waiting around for life to begin or for something to happen in your life, this is a way to create that change. The first act is identifying your trauma, then your needs, wants and values. If you find yourself constantly trying to please others, there is another way to live. You can live authentically and learn to prioritize your needs and achieve your own goals, without fear of alienating yourself from loved ones, in order to live happily and in wholeness. Living fully, freely and authentically according to your own values and pursuing your own dreams is a result of coming into your personal power.

Courage plays a major role in this intense search for self-aware-ness—so much so that it is practically a prerequisite for this book. However, the reward of self-discovery is so great that the toil (and the potential toll—emotional, mental and physical) is worth it. This book is ideal for everyone, from someone with a complete lack of self-awareness to someone who is aware that they have expe-rienced trauma but have no idea why or how it arose. If you have a complete lack of awareness around trauma, it involves how your history has impacted your current emotional state and personal cir-cumstances without your knowledge or understanding (much like yours truly).

In this process, creating awareness requires recalling memo-ries—sometimes painful ones. Journaling will be used to help you clarify your thinking and feeling. Thinking is used as a tool to gen-erate awareness but is not seen as a panacea for solving your prob-lems because of your trauma. Emotion plays a crucial role in this journey, as you will learn. Altering old behaviors and creating new ones, and noticing bodily sensations, play a part in learning about your physical, mental and emotional self, and adapting to different behaviors and attitudes that give you the power to envision and achieve a new life.

ME, YOU AND THE WORK

Although I am a certified counselor in intimate relationships, my acute traumatic response to Myles actually took place *after* the completion of my education. Ironic, no? Or perhaps it is understandable, as I gained some awareness myself in the pro-cess. However, negative social experience has mostly been my teacher because I had what I'd call a life-learning deficit in that my relational experiences were quite limited, due to my temper-ament (shy), social skills (sorely lacking) and upbringing (a lack of interaction and appropriate modeling resulting in trauma from childhood emotional neglect). In my youth, I would never have dreamed of talking to a professional about my issues, had I even recognized them as such. Learning through deduction, it took me a long time to experience my issues in relation to others, and to consequently be able to identify them, because I tended to avoid people. So, if you have trouble dealing with people, I understand, and I wrote this book especially for you.

This book is not meant to replicate traditional "talk" therapy in a clinical setting, and it is based on personal experience gained over a lifetime. Therapy involves exploring experiences in your life and is done in partnership with a counselor or psychologist, which can be of great value. I sought therapy very late in life, and it was an impetus for my education because I wanted to help people, especially those with experiences like mine. If therapy is not the route you want to take, this book offers you a different path—one that worked for me. It is for seekers of truth: your own truth (the only truth that matters, if you ask me). It is for those not afraid of the search, nor, ultimately, of the answers.

It is my sincerest hope for you that by following this path, it may lead you to an awareness of your trauma and its impacts on your life, and to subsequently help you overcome it. The process builds on itself: it starts with a foundation of learning to recognize trauma, thus creating awareness. Next, you build yourself up, brick by proverbial brick. Questions, worksheets, exercises and information in later chapters help you identify, or perhaps even label, your traumatic experience, if helpful, and then seek out the activities that work for you individually so you can heal yourself. Healing work is the best gift you can give yourself. Asking yourself to commit to this work, however difficult, is one of the most loving gestures you can do for you. As you explore your own identity and investigate your emotional triggers to decipher the clues to your trauma, it leads you to seek answers to the questions you may have about yourself.

This book is structured by asking pertinent questions that I ended up asking myself to find answers or explanations for what I was going through. Because I lacked any awareness of my trauma, I started out wondering, *What's wrong with me?* Much later, when I began to understand that the depression I experienced was not, in fact, an inborn trait and not my lot in life, as I had originally thought, I began to wonder, *What happened to me?* I thought about all that I had experienced and determined that it was not "normal" somehow, especially in comparison to others, but I did not know exactly why. I continued the search, and as I gathered answers that resonated with me, I could ask further questions, like *How do I get beyond it?*

As I explored what I had unearthed about myself and my family, I began to wonder, *Can I handle the truth?* I had to reevaluate the influences of both of my parents and reconsider my own thoughts and feelings about myself as I endeavored to change. Once I could accept the possibility that my interpretation of events was also a factor in my trauma, I could see possibilities and potential for my future where I once hadn't been able to, and a new idea emerged: *Can I create a new life for myself?* For me, the answer was a resounding yes, and it can be for you too if you want to take on the challenge of this journey and commit to putting in the work. The next question, naturally, is *How can I do that?* and the strategies and ideas for how to achieve this are made clear later in the book.

A reflective question was next, which is *What have I learned from all of this?* This is the point at which you examine whether you have identified the lessons in your life, informed as it is now by your trauma. Next, you'll ask yourself, *Where do I go from here?* After all, what is this all for, if not for an end result that makes a difference in your life? The final chapter provides reasons for making this commitment to yourself, and for traveling along this path, such as finding your passion and living authentically and happily in wholeness and personal power.

A SENSE OF SELF

My first goal is to bring about a solid sense of self, which is likely to be lacking or missing altogether in each person who has suffered from childhood trauma. Each response to the unique circumstances of a person's childhood is as unique as the person themself. Even though siblings may respond completely differently to a relatively similar upbringing, individuals' reactions vary from person to person, situation to situation and personality to personality. *All* are valid responses. I want to stress this because my sister and I are living examples of it. Each person's experience is their own; the truth for you may not be the same for others, and that is okay. *Your* truth is what matters here; it is just as valid and important as anyone else's.

The part acceptance plays, especially of the self, is paramount. I want you to know that it is possible to get past your trauma and to have a satisfying life. With this book, I hope to help as many people as possible to achieve this for themselves, especially for their own benefit but also for that of their family and beyond into the community. Ultimately, we will have a better world, with a more cohesive society, if the people in it are well adjusted and content. Once you have worked past your emotional triggers, you are powerful indeed, but to get to this point requires work.

COMMIT TO YOURSELF

This process requires your courage, commitment and perseverance, even when it gets tough. Especially when it gets tough, because the avoidance of pain, and denial in particular, creates the worst pain of all. It caused me the greatest emotional devastation, which took the form of the most unspeakable physical pain that I have ever experienced. I truly thought I was going to have a heart attack after realizing that I had wasted not only my own life up to the point of my marital separation but also that of my ex-husband. The guilt and shame of it caused me crushing chest pain. My heart felt like it was in a vise for months. But this was only the beginning of what the unknown, unacknowledged and unaddressed effects of childhood trauma would do to me, as you will see. Yet not only have I survived it but I am thriving. I'm not only here to tell the tale but I'm also grateful for the experiences and the resulting awareness, wholeness and happiness that I achieved, in spite of it all. In guiding you through this process, which was of course my own process, a natural place to start is at the beginning.

Reference

Webb, J. (2012). Dr. Jonice Webb website. Emotional neglect questionnaire. Retrieved (2021) from https://drjonicewebb.com/emotional-neglect-questionnaire/

1

The Start of It All
(And What Is Trauma?)

I HAVE A confession to make: I think I am addicted to drama. I would never have guessed it, but when I look back on my life, especially the last few years, I think I must be, if the way my life has unfolded has told me anything. It sure felt like drama compared to the thirty years preceding it. My new life began, ironically, at a funeral. Technically it was a celebration of life, but funeral just sounds more dramatic (I couldn't help myself). I didn't recognize what was happening at the time, but it felt like a death was occurring inside of me as well on that day. It was the death of my old self and the dawning of a new and better life, if only I had known it at the time.

It was an incredibly large gathering at the service that was held for a friend's brother, who had died one week earlier of a heart attack at a young age. Only three days before his death, I had been at a park with my two children, my friend and her daughter, along with her sister-in-law and her two children. Near the end of our visit on that lovely early spring day, her sister-in-law received a FaceTime call from her husband, whom I'll call Steve. As we pushed our children on the swings, I peeked over her shoulder to get a glimpse of

Steve, whom I had never met or even seen before. Then, three days after his thirty-third birthday, I learned that he was dead. Not only was I utterly shocked, but I was awash with the most eerie feeling that I had ever had. I suppose this was the closest brush with death at a young age that I had ever encountered.

One week later, I attended his celebration of life, which was a beautifully orchestrated and organized event. Many of the family members were musicians who performed touching tributes, and the speeches were poignant, heartfelt, even funny at times. As I sat there among what looked like about a thousand people, a feeling began to creep into my chest. I could feel a strong swelling of emotion, which confused me as I had never even met the man who passed away. I fought valiantly to beat back the tears that were struggling for freedom, but I lost that battle. I was both embarrassed and astounded by my emotional response. By the end of the service, I was sobbing uncontrollably, with makeup running down my cheeks and snot bubbles forming and then dripping down my face, to full dramatic effect. I was a mess. The elderly woman next to me was eyeing me quizzically, perhaps even suspiciously. The only thing that kept me aware of myself and my surroundings was the mortifying idea that people may have thought I was his mistress!

Later, when people were mixing and noshing, I found a hallway near the bathroom and let it all out. It was all I could do just to stay upright. Every time someone went to the washroom, they would look my way in a mix of surprise and sympathy. What was worse was that I was not mourning Steve's passing, but rather experiencing my own sort of passing. Ultimately, this was the start of the passing away of my old life, although I was totally unaware of the meaning behind this event at the time. I did understand, though, that it was of monumental significance, and it would occupy my mind for some time until I came up with answers as to why this had transpired. This mysterious emotional breakdown, which I mustered all of my resources to control, happened regardless. It was simultaneously intense, uncontrolled and protracted, lasting throughout the service and afterward, despite my best efforts to quash it. And it was the best thing to ever happen to me.

At the time I had no idea what was happening, but afterward I wondered about it almost constantly. For months afterward, I would cry myself to sleep each night after Mark had drifted off, not letting him know what I was going through and mystified as to what this meant for my life. I was trying to figure it out on my own. I also had two anxiety attacks, which I had never experienced before. I initially thought that I was grieving for my mother and father, who had each passed away years earlier. And I did grieve for each of them, and for the relationship we never really had (more on that later). Ultimately, I mourned the life I was never allowed to have, or the life I never allowed *myself* to have.

Then, finally, I realized I was also grieving the death of my marriage. I had finally admitted to myself that I was extremely unhappy, and I couldn't see a way to change that within the context of my marriage. It seemed as though my body intelligence had seized the opportunity to issue me a wake-up call in the form of this unexpected breakdown, to get me to pay attention to my needs. It was only because it was something outside myself, that didn't directly affect my life, that the emotional impact of the service was finally able to penetrate my considerable defenses, as I briefly let down my guard.

This is what trauma does to you. It puts up walls to protect you from hurt, but the fear it is based on keeps you from feeling the full extent of the joys and surprises, while also fostering an unyielding angst. It prevents connection and intimacy with other people because it creates a barrier to protect you from what your mind and body perceives as a potential threat of harm. Trauma, especially from the experience of emotional neglect, can be formed over many years, sometimes even decades, stopping your social-emotional development in its tracks and leaving you unequipped to handle adult emotional experience.

It wasn't until recent years that I made sense of what had happened to me to create such unendurable conditions that would prompt me to leave my husband and the life I knew. Due to a lack of social-emotional learning, I was highly influenced by the society around me because I had a limited foundation for forming my own opinions and ideas. Buying a house, renovating it and making babies were what I thought I was *supposed* to do, and were what Mark wanted. Although I was making choices, they weren't based on my own desires. The options that were laid out for me were based on other people's ideas of what was desirable.

As time passed, I began to conceive of having dreams of my own. I remember saying things to myself in the years leading up to my choice to have children, such as *I'm not leading an authentic life.* Instead of paying attention to those misgivings and glimpses of self-knowledge, I doubled down on the people-pleasing aspect of my nature (or nurture, in fact) and convinced myself that doing what would make my husband happy was best because it simply felt like the only real option. My own dreams and desires were just fantasy, and I subjugated them in order to belong.

After the arrival of my first child, I was in full-blown postpartum depression, which was truly miserable. A year after the arrival of my second child, Mark had a serious medical emergency, which was very worrisome and stressful, but fortunately it could be managed with a prescription. However, the way my husband handled the diagnosis (or didn't, more accurately) was the last straw for me. His already-extreme anxiety went through the roof, and it was more than I could handle, with two children, postpartum depression and an as-yet unknown or unrecognized issue lurking in the recesses of my mind. It was only months later that my mental breakdown occurred. One year later, I ended my marriage in a state of complete emotional burnout and utter defeat.

I tore our lives apart because I knew that something had to change. I felt that something was horribly wrong, and I had just barely begun to understand my utter lack of having had my needs met from childhood onwards. It took time for me to figure out that what I was experiencing was personal growth after a prolonged period of stagnation. I was completely unaware of my childhood trauma, and I was only able to put the pieces together after years of attrition removed the outer layers of ignorance, distraction and denial, leaving only the gaping wound at the core. It would be another four years before I healed this core wound using—at various points and over time—the many strategies outlined in this book. My healing took place only after years of subconsciously burying, denying, repressing and eventually numbing my emotions.

It also took me a long time to figure out what had happened in the past to create an environment where my unresolved emotional trauma would eventually explode. I discovered it by revisiting memories from my childhood. It began in the preschool years, when, inexplicably, all physical contact was cut off, with my father in particular, with whom I remember having cuddled in the evenings sometimes. I was never close with my mother, so this taking away of the only love I ever remember receiving was a devastating blow, and I unknowingly spent the rest of my life trying to replace it.

Our "normal" was that we were not a family that said "I love you," and after the preschool years, we did not hug, kiss, cuddle or speak of any feelings whatsoever. Blame it on a stiff-upper-lip British-heritage upbringing, I guess. In fact, I only remember my father saying "I love you" once when I was an adult, when I returned home after disappearing overnight for the first time ever, with no word to anyone, after a particularly demoralizing day at college. It was uncharacteristic of me, to say the least, and is probably the first traumatic response I remember having.

I was the quintessential good girl who always did what I was told, all in an effort to win back my father's love that I had seemingly lost. I never found out why all affection suddenly stopped, and to this day it remains a mystery. I do know that I took after my father, who suffered from depression, disappearing into his room for days at a time, until he reemerged, relatively normal again. My mother, who reacted quickly and sharply during conflict, especially with us children, acted as if nothing were wrong when my father retreated like this, preferring denial as a coping strategy to my father's avoidance, and life carried on. I inherited both of these coping behaviors, dysfunctional as they were.

The effects of trauma only really began to show up in my teen years. My youth was defined by inhibition and detachment, punctuated by bouts of emptiness and despair, as I hid from the world in the privacy of my bedroom. Later, it graduated to raging at the universe and wishing I had never been born. My friends and family knew nothing of my inner life and interpreted my depression as me just being a moody teenager. However, the constant avoidance and denial inevitably devolved into repression, numbing and shutting down emotionally. Self-soothing took the form of going off and being alone, or sleeping endlessly, due to my depression, just as I had learned from my father.

Gradually, as I entered my twenties, I began looking around and noticing differences between myself and my friends. Their relationships with their families were different. My friends were often able to talk to their parents openly, jokingly and even be cheeky sometimes. Their parents, in return, talked to them casually, sometimes teasingly, but generally lovingly, which was foreign to me. This is not to say they were never at odds with their parents, but they had an ease and familiarity in their interactions with their parents that was absent in my household. This became especially apparent when I got into a relationship with my future husband. His family was so *close*. The first time I was hugged by one of his family members, my body went completely rigid. I was not used to such contact. My sister and I were not hugged like that. I don't remember being told as a child by either of my parents that they loved me. I don't even remember them really making much eye contact with me.

WHAT IS TRAUMA?

My definition of trauma is that it is a response to an acute event, or chronic series of events, that you are unable to integrate into your consciousness because it is too painful or is beyond your conscious comprehension. It is often characterized by severe maladaptive coping strategies and overcompensating behaviors like people-pleasing or uncontrolled anger, as well as depression, anxiety and denial. For a more formal definition of trauma, I consulted Merriam-Webster Dictionary Online (2021). In it, trauma is defined as:

1. an injury (such as a wound) to living tissue caused by an extrinsic agent
2. a disordered psychic or behavioral state resulting from severe mental or emotional stress or physical injury
3. an emotional upset

Rhonda Kelloway, a psychotherapist specializing in trauma, defines trauma more simply (2019) as "anything that overwhelms the body's ability to cope. That is, it's too much (or happens too soon or too fast) for you to integrate it physiologically or emotionally," and "anything perceived by the mind or body as life-threatening, leaving you helpless to protect or defend yourself."

Trauma is sometimes only understood as the third definition above. People tend to downplay trauma by confusing a one-time emotional reaction to, say, an angry outburst or verbal assault, with the unconscious effect of compounding emotional stressors over time. We say of that particular moment in time, "I was traumatized," which most certainly can be true, but this can get confused with the long-term effects associated with micro-traumas like emotional neglect. An effect like cPTSD (complex post-traumatic stress disorder) can form, which is more akin to the slow torment of water torture or the small yet pernicious injuries of "death by a thousand cuts," rather than the so-called "flashbacks" typically associated with PTSD. With cPTSD, a layer of trauma is laid down and reinforced each time by the repetition of negative experiences that make you feel unconsciously unworthy, afraid or filled with shame, even if it is an unintentional act on the part of your caregivers.

Although emotional neglect may be considered a lower-grade trauma, that does not make it of lesser significance. It can have a devastating impact on your life, or at least keep you in denial that there is a better, healthier, more integrated life available, due to its ongoing impacts on your thoughts, feelings, behaviors and even bodily sensations. In fact, I would argue that unresolved trauma from emotional neglect in particular, while arguably not the most *detectably* painful experience, is surely the most damaging, especially in terms of socioemotional development and your future mental and emotional state. This was true in my case, since I was neglected by both parents, leaving me emotionally impoverished and unaware of the magnitude of its impact on my nervous system.

The response to the repeated and prolonged wear-and-tear on the body, due to trauma, is called toxic stress syndrome. Harvard University (2021) has this to say about it:

Extensive research on the biology of stress now shows that healthy development can be derailed by excessive or prolonged activation of stress response systems in the body and brain. Such toxic stress can have damaging effects on learning, behavior, and health across the lifespan.

Learning how to cope with adversity is an important part of healthy child development. When we are threatened, our bodies prepare us to respond by increasing our heart rate, blood pressure, and stress hormones, such as cortisol. When a young child's stress response systems are activated within an environment of supportive relationships with adults, these physiological effects are buffered and brought back down to baseline. The result is the development of healthy stress response systems. However, if the stress response is extreme and long-lasting, and buffering relationships are unavailable to the child, the result can be damaged, weakened systems and brain architecture, with lifelong repercussions.

However, it can sometimes be difficult to cobble together the idea of trauma from your unique, if less than ideal, set of experiences, or to form "a case for trauma" for yourself. Reconciling your experience with something as dramatic-sounding as childhood trauma, or the clinical definition above for toxic stress syndrome, may seem far-fetched.

You may feel an inkling of something not being right, but we tend to downplay our emotions, especially if we haven't experienced the horrors of violent abuse. We tell ourselves, *It could be worse*, or we belittle our experience by thinking, *Well, at least I made it out alive.* Sometimes though, we don't want to deal with it, or we don't want to admit it to ourselves. In my case, I simply denied that anything was wrong. I would wallow in self-pity for what I thought was my fate (to be depressed), and mercilessly lambaste myself for my perceived shortcomings (everything from lacking in physical attractiveness to being boring and stupid) in lieu of trying to actually fix the problem, because I didn't rightly know what the problem was. Unfortunately, some people discourage you from talking about your problems because they want to avoid dealing with them themselves. They don't want to hear about it because it reminds them of their own issues, or they may be defensive about their shortcomings as a caregiver.

Family, for example, can sometimes minimize your trauma by saying, "Stop complaining" and advising you to "Get over it," or worse, telling you that it's all in your head, which is a fine example of gaslighting. At the other extreme is the mainstream media and wider society adopting the pop psychology version of trauma, which often focuses on macro-traumas such as the distress experienced by natural disaster survivors, witnesses to a violent crime or the resulting physical and emotional dysfunction of individuals who experienced violent verbal, physical or sexual abuse. What is not as obvious to people and is not focused on in talk shows is that subtle micro-traumas such as emotional neglect, parental separation and divorce or an alcoholic or mentally ill parent are sometimes overlooked because the symptoms are not very obvious and the consequences seem less dire from an outside perspective. However, depending on the situation and the individual's reaction to it, it can be utterly debilitating, especially socially and emotionally.

WHAT TRAUMA CAN LOOK LIKE

Trauma resulting from emotional neglect is an invisible internal injury but is nonetheless real. People who suffer from the effects of it, and whose daily experience is not only affected by it but sometimes even ruled by it, may have experienced emotional blunting, or a marked lack of emotional *expression*, even if their emotions are present and not actually reduced (Cirino, Boland, 2021). They are living a lesser version of life because of their lack of recognition of emotional range and depth. And I know this because this was me.

Trauma can look very different for different people and can be a case of "more than meets the eye." It can show up in overt ways, such as with substance addiction, or it can be very subtle and hide in plain sight with someone who is withdrawn and quiet being labeled as shy when in actuality they are living an emotionally stunted life, which inherently limits their experience, or even impairs their life. In the case of emotional neglect, some people, myself included, thought that they grew up in a relatively "normal" home, ostensibly with parents who loved them. The pain and suffering inflicted is usually unintentional, and the "victims" are usually just as unaware as the "perpetrator" of the effect of the caregiver's negligence. It is likely that some parents have experienced neglect themselves and have simply passed it on. The dysfunction is unrecognized, and the pattern continues.

Dysfunction is a hallmark of trauma, as is suggested by the word itself, which means a lack of proper function. In order to repair the damage and change your life, you must work to get it functioning again, instead of ignoring the issue, hoping it will go away or just accepting it as your "normal." The issue doesn't have to be as obviously severe as something like substance addiction for it to affect you. If trauma has affected your life, it is a big deal, with major potential ramifications and repercussions, even if it seems small and trivial.

Unfortunately, people understand big reactions to big events, but they rarely see or understand responses that are conditioned in us from childhood, that are subtle and ingrained. We may be unaware ourselves of the hole that has been left from the deep impact of trauma, and how it has left scars on our souls. Then, when the festering wound is reopened in adulthood, we react as the child, using the same coping mechanisms we developed in the past, when we sometimes had only ourselves to rely on, with no example set for us by our caregivers. We have little to no ability to effectively self-soothe (calm ourself) in adulthood, because we had no one to support us in the past, leaving us feeling unseen, unheard, unworthy and unloved. Learning to self-soothe is the first step in emotional self-regulation, which is the basis for emotional stability. It bolsters your ability to cope with setbacks and negative experiences. Without this skill, the echoes of the past can return in adulthood to make us repeat the pattern and relive the unrecognized hurts of childhood.

As children, we are (usually) dependent on adult caregivers to feed and shelter us. In the absence of adults providing these necessities as well as loving care and attention, a child is constantly in survival mode, displaying whatever behaviors or doing whatever it takes to get their needs met. Children in this situation instinctually respond to everything that is perceived as a threat to their safety and security through the fight/flight/freeze/fawn—also known as the fight/flight/freeze/appease—response in order to cope. The greater the number of traumatic experiences, the greater the impact of trauma on the individual, contributing to a whole host of psychological, emotional and sometimes even physical problems. As I discovered, my reactions were to flee (flight), to appease (fawn) and sometimes even to freeze, all of which kept me from experiencing authentic interactions within my relationships. To me, the most tragic result of trauma is the inability to connect with others. Not learning this skill in childhood has haunted me into adulthood and is hard to correct, particularly if you are unaware.

I kept wondering what differed between me and other people when interacting. I became a people-watcher, trying to discern the nuances of people relating and talking. I hadn't learned basic communication skills because I didn't have communicative parents. I was socially inept, and the ease with which people conversed was such a mystery to me. This fascination is probably why I ended up in counseling psychology. Over thirty years I had learned a thing or two, so eventually, and for the first time, I was able to put to work the skills I had slowly learned by going out and making new friends, which is a bit nerve-racking in your forties, let me tell you.

Every situation will vary, and each person's experience is unique, so yours will probably be completely different from my situation, in both how you think and feel about it. Factors such as your personality, your temperament, your family situation and the level of stress in your life can affect individuals in many different ways. If you have instances of anxiety, insecurity or the inability to deal with stress effectively, especially without an obvious source, you may find yourself being judged for your actions or reactions, and being viewed as weak by others. You may even feel weak yourself! I have seen people who seek to please others ad nauseam break down in tears at the slightest affront, or constantly strive for perfection. Others, like me, have numbed themselves to the point that they have shut down emotionally and have shut people out.

THE FIRST STEP

Acknowledging your trauma is the first step, whether it was from transgressions made against you or an unintentional lack of regard for you. If you discount or dismiss what you experienced, you truly do yourself a disservice. I was forced to acknowledge that things were irretrievably and irrevocably changed after my emotional breakdown at that funeral, since it happened so publicly and unexpectedly. What had started out as an utter mystery to me about the origins of my reaction began to make sense as I delved deeper into not only what could have preceded it but also what could have *predisposed* me to it.

It was a slow realization about how my life was different from others around me. It was not that my parents were overly strict or authoritarian (except for my father, on rare occasions of severe physical punishment). Actually, they were both quite uninvolved and seemingly apathetic. The behaviors that had manifested in me, such as dissociation and withdrawal, were definitely unnoticed by my parents, or else they were just not seen as being a problem. Most days, I felt invisible. It was the lack of interaction, attention, affection and belonging, plus an apparently uncaring attitude of indifference, that left such an indelible imprint on my soul.

The removal of physical touch at such a young age created an overwhelming sense of abandonment. It also created an all-encompassing fear of emotional intimacy which impaired my ability to bond in a healthy way. As a teenager and young adult, even while in a relationship, I constantly and compulsively sought validation from others (being noticed, or "seen" by men), since I never got it from my parents. Eventually, I unconsciously numbed myself to protect myself from the pain of realizing how evidently unimportant I was. All this resulted in me having a profound lack of self-worth, self-love and self-acceptance because I felt unworthy of love. I hated myself. Most of the time, I wished I weren't there. I was a stranger to myself, and I felt like an outsider in my own family. It left me always seeking, even feeling obligated, to please others just for any scrap of attention. Ultimately, it led to me forgoing my own needs and desires to live someone else's dream. I've finally woken up from that dream to create ones of my own.

NEXT STEPS

I offer you practical steps to achieve your own revelations as well, no matter where you are in life. Whatever the circumstances in which you may find yourself, it is important to always know that it is possible to change them. It really, *really* may not feel like it, but when it comes down to it, it's always a matter of choice. Even at my lowest point, something made me hang on. I had some inner reserve of strength that I didn't know I possessed, allowing me to see possibilities that I couldn't see previously, and this realization informed me that change was possible. However, to turn possibilities into reality can sometimes take considerable time and effort.

As the structure of the book suggests, I began my own work by looking at my life and questioning. I began investigating the source of my problems, but before that, I had to ask myself whether I was living the life I wanted. It took me a long time to admit that the answer was no. I felt I had to justify it somehow, probably because I was so used to waiting for permission from others, so I had to learn to decide for myself what was best. This was something new for me. After overcoming the initial roadblocks of allowing myself to do the work, I began thinking deeply about what brought me to where I was. I pored over my life situation, my memories and my personality traits in search of answers, and I made some surprising discoveries, based on my own intuition. You will use your intuition in the same way.

The work involves making connections between what may have occurred in your past with the current condition of your psyche. It involves bringing what isn't currently known mentally, emotionally and possibly even physically (for example, an unexplained ache or pain) to the forefront so that it can be identified, labeled (if helpful to you), fully explored and felt, perhaps for the first time. This can be achieved through various means, including some exercises that will be presented so you can practice experiencing emotions and processing sensations. Trauma can then be integrated into your life as experience rather than being seen as a tragedy that stops you from living.

It is not my intention for you to re-traumatize yourself by revisiting and reliving past torment. I did all of these things safely, in search of answers, and the fortunate side effect was the integration I experienced by reflecting on all the events of my life and coming to awareness about myself. These exercises, practices and strategies are meant to bring about awareness in the body as well as using your mind to help you identify trauma and process the information you glean from your history rather than to relive the moment.

Trauma doesn't need to maintain its grip on your life. The idea is to understand, accept and deal with its overwhelmingly life-changing effects by dealing with the aftermath of that experience, but also to *alter* your response and perhaps even your *perception* of that experience. Becoming aware and identifying your trauma is the path to wholeness in this process. Happiness is achieved by accepting what happened, letting go of expectations of yourself and others, then simply letting life's events unfold for you in an organic way. Integration is the key to the personal power aspect of this work.

These things combined provide the basis for learning who you truly are, free from interference from others. Then you can find out what motivated you to act as you did, make the choices you made and react the way you did. It all starts with awareness. This in turn can provoke self-discovery about what you really want from life and what lights a fire inside you. Let your intuition guide you toward your passion and allow you to see, perhaps for the first time, a way forward—from undefined desperation and despair to living with intention and passion. From trauma to triumph.

Chapter 1 References

Merriam-Webster (2021). Merriam-Webster Dictionary Online. Trauma definition. Retrieved (2021) from https://www.merriam-webster. com/dictionary/trauma

Kelloway, R. (2019). LifeCare Wellness blog. "3 ways childhood trauma can affect your adult relationships." Retrieved (2020) from https://life-care-wellness.com/3-ways-childhood-trauma-can-affect-your-adult-relationships/

Harvard University (2021). Center on the Developing Child online. "Toxic stress: Key Concepts." Retrieved (2021) from https:// developingchild.harvard.edu/science/key-concepts/toxic-stress/

Cirino, E., & Boland, M. (2021). Healthline. "Recognizing emotional blunting and finding help." Published May 13, 2021. Retrieved (2021) from https://www.healthline.com/health/mental-health/emotional-blunting#takeaway

2

Becoming Aware:
What's Wrong with Me?

THE MAIN FOCUS of this chapter is getting you to learn about yourself, which is ultimately in service of identifying your trauma. If you lack awareness, like I did, about the experiences that led to your current state of dissatisfaction or disempowerment, the first question that naturally arises (as it did for me) is "What's wrong with me?" It's a start, but we need to dig down into how you are actually feeling. The following questions that I asked myself may apply for you as well. Do you have a vague sense of unhappiness, uneasiness, dissatisfaction, lack of fulfillment or perhaps even imbalance in your life? Are you often left wondering, waiting for your chance, or waiting for permission to begin your life? Perhaps you have always felt obligated to fulfill other people's wants, forgoing your own needs and desires. Perhaps you are always striving, always working toward that elusive goal, believing that once there, only then you will feel like you are "somebody," or that you will feel worthy.

Often you don't allow yourself to pursue things for fear of disapproval from your partner or family, especially if it will impinge on their expectations of you or offend your own sense of duty. It can leave you feeling empty and devoid of meaning. However, not pursuing your goals, if you even have any idea of what those are, is easier than disappointing others. If you feel guilt or shame about what it is that you want out of life, and you believe that pursuing your own dreams may disrupt your relationships, this response is a red flag. Feeling unworthy of time to yourself or denying your own desires is indicative of an overall lack of self-love and self-worth, which comes with this kind of trauma. Over time, if unresolved, it can leave you at risk for sinking into a deep yet inexplicable state of despair and depression, or possibly even contemplating suicide, without an apparent cause or an obvious source of your pain.

If you always put others' needs ahead of your own, not only because you love them and want to take care of them but because you feel obligated to do so, or you do things that you *think* are what someone else wants, your low self-worth may have manifested in you becoming a pleaser. If you're always saying yes to others' requests or agreeing with them for fear of offending them and creating conflict, sparking anxiety and an unconscious fear that the person will leave or abandon you, this is likely a traumatic response. If you find you are compromising yourself to please a partner or family member, you may be codependent or possibly enmeshed with that person due to your traumatic experience.

The difference between these concepts is that enmeshment is a situation with two people who have unclear boundaries in their emotional relationship, whereas codependency is a relationship dynamic with one person enabling the other; either one can have trauma as a source of the issue. I was in a codependent relationship with Mark because I put my needs secondary to his desires, which were driven by his anxiety. He was enmeshed with me, however, because he envisaged us as a single entity or unit, which not only easily translated to having no unique identities of our own, but was also handily enabled and supported by my codependency issues. Until I realized there was an alternate way to live, I allowed this to continue for most of our relationship because I didn't know any better, nor did I know how else to maintain our relationship.

LEARNING ABOUT TRAUMA

One evening in 2018, I stumbled upon the concept of childhood trauma (and specifically the Adverse Childhood Experiences questionnaire, which I will get to later in this chapter), just by talking randomly to someone at a nightclub that I frequented. That one bit of information set me on a path of personal inquiry, investigation and discovery of my trauma, which was extremely helpful, and it highlights a vital reason for pursuing things that are important to you (such as dancing was for me). You never know who you might meet who could change the course of your life. Shortly before that time, I had also met someone else at that club who would permanently and irreversibly alter my life's trajectory.

I'll never forget the moment I laid eyes on Myles. I felt like I had been struck by lightning. I even said out loud to myself, "Wow!" as I stood there, awestruck, trying to regain my composure and the strength in my knees. I was electrified by my attraction for him, and I was instantly infatuated. But it was more than that. It was the most powerful experience of my life, and I almost immediately recognized it for what it was: a soul connection. I felt a sense of *knowing* that this was the person I wanted to be with, like ... for life. Call it what you want: "love at first sight," passion or what the French call "jouissance."

Myles was the most extraordinary person (and, full disclosure, the sexiest man) I had ever met. I was extremely attracted and drawn to him, and I know that he was to me as well. We were both hopelessly shy and socially awkward, however. Despite this, each time we saw each other at the club, we found a nonverbal way to communicate, with smoldering looks and smiles. Though our conversations were short and superficial as we struggled to break through the impasse to something more meaningful, it more often than not left me wanting more despite the difficulty. We were both experts at covertly observing one another, getting to know each other by proxy and watching our interactions with others. We very much liked each other from what we had witnessed. Perhaps it was the atmosphere of the club, with the lights and the music, plus these tantalizing interactions, however brief and lacking in critical information about each other, but in no time, I had fallen deeply in love with him. However, he triggered me like no one else ever could.

RECOGNIZING TRAUMA

Struggling to connect the scattered and seemingly unrelated dots of your life in order to discern the cause of your issues can be the most frustrating part of this inquiry into the self. As you can see, problems with relationships can be one of the biggest indicators. If you are unable to form romantic relationships because you are afraid to be vulnerable, especially of loving someone so much that you are afraid of losing them, this could be indicative of abandonment issues in childhood, as in my example, which stems from my relationship with my father. This person who you care for so deeply has likely tapped into that former trauma. Only the threat of a loss of that magnitude can create such a fear response. Trust me on that one.

I was astonished that it was possible to feel that way about someone, especially since Myles and I were never together as a couple. Unfortunately, unconscious fear kept me—and I suspect him too—from allowing us to get close. Our guards were always up, and we would constantly trigger each other, but especially me. I didn't even know what "triggering" meant until much later. All I knew was that I seemed to be fighting myself when I went to talk to him. It was maddening. As time passed, it sometimes got so bad that I couldn't say one word in response to him. It was frustrating for him and humiliating for me. It felt truly tragic.

The first time I had a traumatic response to him, I didn't even know what it was. Over the weeks that we first saw each other at the hang out where I went dancing with my friends, despite the lingering looks of obvious attraction between us, the first time Myles came up to talk to me, after brief introductions, I felt something click in my head and I immediately walked away, leaving a trail of confusion in my wake. Little did I know that he had triggered my fight/flight/freeze/fawn response. I was as bewildered as he was, as I had never felt that before, and I began to obsessively question what that moment meant. I had to come up with answers using my own resources, which is what I will be guiding you to do.

LOOKING FOR CONNECTIONS

What you will be reading here is different from traditional forms of counseling psychology, or talk therapy, because you are doing the work by yourself, with only your supports to help you. I will give you specific things to think about as well as some exercises to do later in this chapter. Mostly it requires you to remember, think and feel, but in a different way. The goal is to use memories to gain access to insight. This will allow you to make connections between your past and your current situation, access to which may have been cut off many years ago. I am asking you to search your memories for situations that stand out and record them in a journal. The reason that this is important is that the most memorable events of your life have a particular emotional impact, or perhaps even a lack thereof, and those are the points at which you can make connections. I recalled only a few key memories myself but enough to help this process work. It is by remembering and thinking about the emotions that were felt, or seemingly not felt, that you can begin to grasp the impact and relevance of those emotional reactions. It is also useful to note the times you did not react and what that meant.

You can also use others' reactions as a guide for the times when you did not react but other people did, and ask yourself why that is. It is not the point to compare yourself to others and to judge their reaction as somehow better. It is just a useful gauge when you are struggling to see how things affected you in the past. Think of it as simply observing differences instead. Did you freeze when others reacted? You can compare your response to theirs to discover information, rather than use it as another source of shame or reason for self-reproach. You're not here for that. Use the information you discover to help you instead. Bringing up old memories can help you uncover patterns that will guide you to make intuitive connections among all the things that have contributed to your situation now. You can begin to connect the reasons for why these memories are so important with what they represented to you in childhood. This shows you how you reacted and responded. Remember that not responding is also a response. Then try to recall how you felt at that time.

How you feel about that situation now, with your adult thinking and experiences to guide you, can be used as a way to find the emotional triggers that are there but were never recognized by you as a child or as an adult until you noticed the patterns that have negatively impacted your life. As I explain below, you are examining your reaction in order to see if you can remember how you felt back then, without judgment, and identifying the emotions, rather than reliving them. This can give you clues about your reaction to the situation and how it arose, but you may have some difficulty with this task.

AVOIDANCE OF PAIN

Our natural tendency is to try to avoid pain. It is an actual evolutionary function to aid in the survival of the species, by avoiding accidents that can threaten our lives. The avoidance of pain is rooted in fear. According to Alexis Wnuk (2021), science writer and editor for BrainFacts.org, "Our brains are hardwired for fear—it helps us identify and avoid threats to our safety. The key node in our fear wiring is in the amygdala, a paired, almond-shaped structure deep within the brain involved in emotion and memory." In our modern context we still seek to actively avoid suffering, even though physical threats to our existence (like the sabertooth tiger) no longer exist, and this can be our undoing. Often what we are now avoiding is psychological stress, which the body has internalized as a real-life threat, by conflating it with our conditioning from childhood emotional neglect because we rely on our parents or caregivers for survival. So, if I were to ask you to go whip up your most painful memory, and you find yourself at this point wanting to put the book down and get up to go change those lightbulbs that have been burnt out in the ceiling fan for years, it is an understandable reaction.

We tend to do this in many aspects of our lives. If we don't want to deal with it, we will find some way, any way, to busy ourselves, distract ourselves and avoid at all costs doing that which has the potential to cause us emotional pain, or any pain really. It is no wonder if you are having difficulty with this task. This is what you have tried to avoid, and for good reason. To intentionally go back to your most painful memories and retrieve them for inspection, and to risk reexperiencing them in some way, sounds like a fast track to re-traumatizing yourself. Obviously, this is not the point of what I am asking you to do. In my experience, it is possible to remember what happened without revisiting that moment in time. It was not retrieving memories that re-traumatized me, but rather trauma reenactment, which is unlikely in this scenario. It may seem risky, but to not attend to your past in this way risks much more: you will not learn and grow from your past experiences.

Developing your awareness is paramount to your success in this quest. This is where your courage comes into play—but also your self-interest. It's better to know than to deny the truth, and it's better to change than to remain stuck. Try thinking of it this way: I am asking you to grab your pipe and magnifying glass, put your Sherlock Holmes hat on, and attentively and *objectively* look at the circumstances surrounding your trauma. The point is to remember and identify *what* you felt, rather than trying to reexperience *how* it felt. Get curious and become your own detective, searching for ancient clues on the trail back to your childhood, to the scene of the crime, as it were. I did this intensively, with no emotional ill effects, and it helped me answer some of my own questions, after which I slowly and deliberately dealt with the emotional aftermath of the discoveries.

For me, contending with the meaning of those memories was the hard part. However, do keep in mind that retrieving memories could potentially be painful for some, because everyone's experience is unique and their ability to cope is different. Finding the relevant memories, evaluating their effect on you and connecting the events to one another is what will help you define your trauma, plus learning to feel in general, if you have lacked in this area, as I did, is the key to unlocking your freedom from trauma. Try to keep in mind the reward for your efforts. You are finding *yourself*! The reward is ultimately to make your life better.

The added bonus of this strategy of learning to detect your trauma is to stimulate your insight and develop your intuition. Do you "trust your gut," or does your heart guide you? If you are unsure, do a self-check, from an embodiment perspective, for where emotion is felt in you. Where in your body can you feel it affect you, not just from your childhood experiences, but generally speaking in your adult life? Did you ever get a "sick" feeling from something? How about a sensation of sadness? Or love? Has anyone ever jumped out and scared you? Where in your body did you feel a reaction? These questions may help you get in touch with your emotions, but more importantly, they may also help you attune yourself to your body. Recognizing an emotion and sensing where you feel it in your body is an important step in learning how it impacts you, as well as what it is telling you. A lot of trauma can be trapped in the body in the form of aches and pains, stiffness or other medical issues. This can be a result of stuffing down the emotions and repressing them in response to trauma.

Sometimes memories can be foggy, and the time you are recalling was too long ago to remember the feeling, or you just may not be able to discern any emotional reaction, even if you do have memories. You may be able to use an "appropriate" or understandable emotion as a placeholder, because your reaction may have been much more subtle than you realize. It took me a long time to interpret how I was reacting, as an adult, to the abandonment I felt as a child. My biggest clue was the fact that I was always a "good girl." I avoided behaviors that would get me into trouble from my parents at all costs. I repressed any emotions that were "unbecoming of a young lady," particularly anger, so I was unable to recognize the emotion, or at least connect it to those rare occasions of expressing my seething rage while alone in my bedroom. As an adult, I finally realized that losing my father's love was an act of betrayal that left me hurt and angry, especially since I couldn't figure out *why* I had apparently lost his love. I felt as though I was "not allowed" to get angry as a child, so finding a placeholder emotion as an adult for what I thought I "should" have felt back then was essential to unlocking my trauma. That's how I was able to make the connection.

MY OWN MEMORIES

My most impactful memory was when I was a preteen and I complained to my father about something by saying, "It's not fair!" He then said, in an unsympathetic tone, "Who said life was fair?" This may seem rather harmless from an outside perspective, but for me, it was life-altering. As a preschooler, I felt abandoned by him, as well as the distinct loss of love from the first and foremost man of importance in my life, and perhaps for the first time since then, I had felt safe enough to complain to him. I not only felt betrayed by his lack of empathy and caring, but it also cemented my trauma from earlier on. There was no recognition of my efforts to be a "good girl" for all those years. There was no reward.

What I learned from that experience onward was that he didn't have my back. Nobody did. I internalized that I was truly alone and that no one could be trusted. I didn't actually recognize these things as feelings. I didn't have the awareness or the practice to feel anything at all. The only way that I had learned to cope was to repress. It was after this time that I began to sink into what would become years of chronic depression. To some it may seem that I was overly sensitive, and perhaps I was a sensitive child. I know my parents were well intentioned, and they did look after my physical needs. I recognize that they did the best they could with the skills, knowledge and understanding that they had at the time. I do know that they loved me, at least now; however, their lack of attunement to my emotional state (of being so withdrawn) and their lack of attention to my emotional needs provided the basis for what was to become of my adult life.

Even though parents likely never mean to injure their child in this way, it is up to them to notice the child's behavior in order to foster a healthy sense of well-being. The way a child internalizes their experience is a factor that can't be accounted for by parents alone, but they can *respond* to their child's behaviors. Children simply do not have the developmental capacity to question their caregivers and therefore, out of necessity, they blindly accept the level of care offered and the example set by their parents. At their early level of development and lack of experience, children are dependent on and beholden to the experience their parents bestow upon them. It is up to the adult, the parent, to attune to their children's physical *and* emotional needs at least one-third of the time to be effective parents (Kelloway, 2019). It can mean the difference between overall health and well-being and a lifelong mental and socioemotional struggle.

I was a textbook case of arrested psychological development, which means that my development literally stopped. My social and emotional learning was absent throughout childhood and adolescence, resulting in difficulty with emotional and verbal expression, and even some cognitive deficits, especially in the application of skills. I didn't actually think about my experience; therefore, I had no insight. I had only ever learned to react, relying solely on instinct, not knowing any other way to perceive. Left to my own devices, I turned inward, repressing all emotion, while my sister turned outward, expressing full-blown rebellion by constantly sneaking out at night, drinking heavily, experimenting with all sorts of drugs and being promiscuous. She was pretty much completely out of control, while I was the polar opposite. Honestly, I wish I had been more like her, because at least she got some of her needs met.

WHO CAN YOU TURN TO?

If you have experienced emotional neglect from both parents, as I did, the only saving graces at this point, with a lack of parental support, are in your external circumstances, such as your friends, other family members, clergy or other religious affiliates, perhaps even teachers, coaches, school counselors, or other community support workers such as youth workers or community center staff. We are a social species, and without proper support we have gaps in socioemotional learning that have a persistent, overarching negative effect on our lives.

DON'T GO IT ALONE

Going it alone on this journey has major disadvantages. It can leave you vulnerable to distortion and minimizing your problems. Part of my problem was not recognizing my supports, because my trust was so broken and my self-image so poor that I thought I would be bothering people if I asked for help, had I known how to do that or even recognized the need for it. I felt alone in my experience and believed I was of no importance to anyone.

Many times, people suffer alone, unaware of their suffering as suffering, and accepting what fate has dealt them, not realizing that there is any alternative. This is why making these connections is so important if you have suffered in silence, ignorant of your own needs and impotent to secure any sense of control over your life. You may be riddled with feelings of worthlessness that you believe are an innate rather than a learned trait. This is what tugs at my heartstrings, because I was like this. This book is for those lost souls who escaped everyone's notice, or were ignored, never having their silent struggle acknowledged, their pain recognized—even by themselves—nor their tragic, shrunken experience. Those traumatized individuals have difficulty with the concept of being entitled to take up space in the world, let alone having a good life.

You may not think you are worth the effort that others want to put in, but please deny the impulse to shut out the people who love you. Seek support wherever you can. The people in your life can listen, console and comfort you, or help you find resources if you need help. It can be as simple as a hug from a loved one or a sit-down conversation to communicate what you need from your partner, family member or a friend. Maybe they can take care of the kids while you try to work on yourself. Try to express that you are going through something big and getting their aid will help you. Then tell them how and what would be of most help. Start small. You can choose to involve other people, professional or not, but taking advantage of the supports you already have is so beneficial to your journey, if for no other reason than to feel, receive and maintain human connection.

ADVERSE CHILDHOOD EXPERIENCES

Another way to narrow down the search is to take the Adverse Childhood Experiences survey, which uses ten areas of childhood trauma that were identified in a 1995 study on obesity that was conducted with 286 participants by Kaiser Permanente, a Health Maintenance Organization in the United States (CDC, 1995). It was later followed up in 1997 with the Centers for Disease Control using data from 17,337 volunteers, because the findings of the original study indicated a large proportion of people with obesity dropped out of the weight loss program, despite success, as they had experienced sexual abuse as children. The sexual abuse reported by these people correlated with their drop-out rate. This indicated that trauma was much more common than the researchers had realized. The combined results of these studies were named the Adverse Childhood Experience study (ACEs) and were developed into a scale to identify these experiences. The basic scale includes ten areas of trauma, but the more comprehensive scale of 200 questions addresses much more specific, and much less recognized, causes of trauma (CDC, 1997). Either can be used to help identify traumas that you may be unaware of. I scoured the 200 questions, and it was just one singular question that showed me the "symptom" that alerted me to the fact that I had been emotionally neglected, because I had no understanding of it otherwise.

These are the ten areas that were most commonly identified in the Kaiser Permanente study. There are five personal types of childhood trauma: physical abuse, verbal abuse, sexual abuse, physical neglect and emotional neglect. The other five types are related to other family members such as an alcoholic parent, a mother who is a victim of domestic violence, a family member who is in jail, a family member diagnosed with a mental illness and the disappearance of a parent through divorce, death or abandonment (Aces Too High, 2020). There is also a resiliency questionnaire to help you determine what supports, if any, you may have been able to access and benefit from. However, if you struggle to identify your trauma, awareness can still come from internal sources, as it did for me, using my memories as a resource. Using my strategy as a guide, you can make those connections if your trauma is not clear to you, yet you recognize that something was undoubtedly very wrong in your childhood.

Memory Retrieval Exercise

This was the first conscious step I took in trying to work out how my past had impacted me. Using this exercise I created, think back to some of your earliest memories. Are they happy? Perhaps some are and some are not. Perhaps none are. Whatever they are, try to remember those that seem foremost in your mind. Really consider why that is so. What about that memory holds a certain value or quality to it? What is that quality? Is it sadness, anger, loneliness, shock, panic or fear? Is it anxiety, due to your helplessness and dependence on this adult or even full-blown betrayal, abandonment or neglect? Are you able to detect this from your memory? Or is it something more nuanced that you can't quite identify? Whatever it is, do your best to record it in a journal. Continue recording any other memories and their emotional content as well.

If there are no memories that you can think of, are there any situations, behaviors or events that seem to repeat in your history, whether it is your or your family member's actions? What are they? Searching for patterns helps you discover the source from which your coping behaviors developed. This is in no way suggesting that thinking your way out of trauma is the answer. Your feelings, sensations and behaviors are also relevant aspects to examine in yourself, but that comes later in the process. This is only a tool to help you discover patterns in your and your family's history in order to discern how your upbringing has shaped your life. You can make connections as to why you reacted, or perhaps didn't, to the ways your caregivers interacted with you, even if you never noticed anything before. This simply is your M.O. I certainly was able to determine mine, as in the "good girl" example.

If you experience an overwhelming emotional reaction from your memory, and you are unable to continue, stop immediately. Go to the breathing and grounding exercises below. However, if you are able to continue, do attempt to identify the feeling and include that in your journal. If you trigger an emotion, try to sit with it, just for a second or two. If you can, locate where you are feeling it in your body. Record this in your journal as well. If at any time this is too much for you, abandon the exercise for now. The point is not to re-traumatize you. If you sense that you are unable to handle the level of emotion being brought up by the memory retrieval exercise, follow the breathing and grounding exercises below to bring you back to the present moment. If you feel that you can, try again. If not, you can try this at a later time, in the chapter where I guide you to sit with your emotions.

Breathing Exercise

Sit comfortably, with eyes closed. Breathe in through the nose for six seconds, hold for one second, then breathe out through the mouth for eight seconds. Repeat as many times as is comfortable, until you feel calm. This helps release built-up tension and gets you to focus on your breath when the pain seeps in. It helps to expand your chest and lungs when they want to contract in reaction to your painful memories. If you find yourself ruminating about the memories you have brought up, use the following grounding exercise to mindfully return to the present moment.

Grounding Exercise

Sit comfortably on the floor if possible (use a cushion if you want) with legs crossed, or in a kitchen-type chair, in order to keep your back upright and not slouching. Close your eyes and keep your hands on top of your thighs, or turn your hands upward with the palms up. Notice the floor under your seat and legs, or if in a chair, the floor under your feet. Notice the weight in the seat of your chair, and feel how supported you are by it and the earth underneath it. Notice the temperature of the air as you breathe in and out in a slow, rhythmic fashion, but keep it natural and relaxed, not forced. Breathe in and out through your nose, but if you need to, breathe out through your mouth. Notice the sensation of your skin against the fabric of your clothes and the air on the areas of exposed skin. Pay attention to your surroundings now. Can you hear birds or traffic outside your window? Can you hear the hum of the fridge? Can you smell anything in your surroundings? Paying attention to these things brings you into the present moment while allowing you to focus on yourself and your bodily sensations. You may also notice interior feelings. Is there tightness in your chest? Is your stomach clenched? Are your muscles relaxed or tight? The common response to pain is to contract and tighten. Focus on any tight areas and try to get them to relax or unclench, while breathing and counting as in the first exercise, and then release the breath through your mouth.

Chapter 2 References

Wnuk, A. (2021). BrainFacts/SfN. *The root of fear and anxiety.* BrainFacts.org. November 27, 2016. Retrieved (2021) from https://www.brainfacts.org/thinking-sensing-and-behaving/emotions-stress-and-anxiety/2016/image-of-the-week-the-root-of-fear-and-anxiety-110716

Kelloway, R. (2019). LifeCare Wellness blog. *3 ways childhood trauma can affect your adult relationships.* Retrieved (2020) from https://life-care-wellness.com/3-ways-childhood-trauma-can-affect-your-adult-relationships/

CDC (1995). Centers for Disease Control and Prevention website. *About the CDC-Kaiser ACE study.* Violence Prevention. Retrieved

(2020) from https://www.cdc.gov/violenceprevention/aces/about.html?CDC_AA_refVal=https%3A%2F%2Fwww.cdc.gov%2Fviolenceprevention%2Facestudy%2Fabout.html

CDC (1997). Centers for Disease Control and Prevention website. *Adverse Childhood Experiences (ACEs)*. Violence Prevention. Retrieved (2020) from https://www.cdc.gov/violenceprevention/aces/index.html?CDC_AA_refVal=https%3A%2F%2Fwww.cdc.gov%2Fviolenceprevention%2Facestudy%2Findex.html

AcesTooHigh (2020). Aces Too High News. *Got your ACEs score?* Retrieved (2020) from https://acestoohigh.com/got-your-ace-score/

3

Building Resilience:
What Happened to Me?

IN THE LAST chapter, I introduced you to the idea that, like me, you may not have even realized that you have a problem. Once you do, though, you may have questions. The next question I found myself asking was, *What happened to me?* I continued later with, *How did I end up like this? What was the chain of events that led to me being like this, and now that I have come to awareness, what comes next? How do I move from awareness into healing?* Building resilience is the next step in the process.

Continuing from the last chapter, I will build on the memory retrieval exercise, using a new exercise, plus others I will explain later on, to shore up your resilience by learning to feel again. Consult your journal to look at the memories that stood out for you, and which emotion you felt at the time, if anything. If you didn't record anything because you couldn't detect an emotion for that event, you could interview family, such as siblings (which I did), to see what their memories and experience of certain situations and events were, or what growing up was like in general. This may or may not be helpful. For instance, if siblings interpreted things completely differently or had opposing experiences to yours, they may try to convince you that you were wrong. Even if you don't fill them in on why you are inquiring, they may catch on and criticize you in your endeavor. If you're not prepared for this, their disapproval may hinder your progress this early on in the process.

There are other tactics that may be less emotionally risky. In the past, you may have used other coping mechanisms to avoid any overwhelming emotions, such as distracting yourself with overeating, drinking alcohol or using substances. You may have denied your feelings and maintained "a stiff upper lip," as I did, rationalizing that if you can just "keep it together," everything will be fine. If you don't remember feeling any emotion at all, having suppressed all feelings or perhaps dissociating ("going to your happy place"), try to imagine what would be the "appropriate" emotion. Alternatively, if you were telling a friend about that memory, how do you think they would react? What would they say to you? Do words like *horrible*, *terrible* or *sad* come to mind? Let your imagination guide you.

Perhaps, if it feels safe to do so, you could actually tell a friend about your experiences and get a real reaction to your story. Seeing how others react can provide clues if you are struggling to even identify what emotion you experienced, or suppressed, let alone figure out what event may have created your traumatic response. Sometimes, something someone else says can ring true, even if you don't remember feeling it, but it fits intellectually with what you've pieced together about these situations from childhood, which serves to illuminate how they so greatly impacted your adult life.

Once you connect the dots for yourself—by looking at your upbringing, your relationships, your reactions or responses—and you start to identify what happened to you, you can begin the process of doing something about it. Learning your reactions to the situation is one of the more difficult aspects of this work, because it can be hard enough just to identify your trauma, so your first instinct is to blame your parents or whomever for whatever harm they apparently caused you. In the case of overt abuse, then yes, it is obvious that they harmed you. However, there are other instances where you may have internalized a version of events that differed from the actual event, or attached feelings to or thoughts about an event that are not accurate.

LEARNING FROM THE PAST

In my case of emotional neglect, I only discovered as an adult that my parents failed to provide me almost any emotional support or even a feeling of being loved; however, I did understand intellectually that this was not their intent, and that they loved me but did not know how to show it. Having internalized certain reactions to their behavior (such as appeasing them in order to stay on their good side, although never feeling "good enough" and never allowing my own sense of self to develop) is what led to my feelings of unworthiness and seeking external validation through the attention of men. My husband, Mark, whom I met at 16, provided the perfect emotional backdrop to reinforce my "daddy issues."

When we were teenagers, Mark was insecure and wanted me to cast off my old friendships and move into his world, which I did because I was such a pleaser. We formed this incredibly insular partnership, with no individual identities of our own. It's no surprise to me that I was drawn to this person, as his anxious tendencies found a perfect match to my level of avoidance. His anxieties made him want to control my behaviors, which made me emotionally retreat. He would demand pledges of love, which I was barely able to provide, and this made him more anxious. I was afraid of his reactions, because it meant I was constantly on the defense, trying to appease him. The demands placed on me and the constant pressure to "perform" made me avoidant. Eventually I would just shut down and stay silent.

I was unable to communicate and, consequently, I was unable to ask for what I needed in the relationship. I was unaware that I even had needs, other than sexual ones, because I had lived without them being recognized by anyone for so long—including me—and there was definitely no recognition of them on his part either. I often felt invalidated by the one phrase, "You don't really think that, do you?" I felt unseen, as in my childhood, which provided the stimulus for me to seek attention elsewhere.

However, Mark was my security. He was a replacement for my father, and I immediately began the same pattern of trying to do what I thought he wanted. I was a pleaser in order to maintain his affection for me. It was a recipe for disaster as he was a pleaser too, albeit an anxious one, who vacillated between making demands and trying to appease. It took decades before I began to understand and had finally defined for myself that I was not living according to my own desires, nor my own values, such as the freedom to do, say and think whatever I wanted, as well as to enjoy my right to alone time.

Trying to please someone else, while I had begun to grow and learn, bit by bit, over time, brought me to an impasse. I was still following the script I learned from childhood about how to get love from someone. Only I wasn't able to return that love in a meaningful way, although I tried. Mark constantly asked me if I loved him, and I would say yes, to please him, instead of being motivated by my real feelings of love. The tactic had the exact opposite effect of what he intended. It pushed me further away. I didn't know how to supply him with the love and affection he demanded so often and so vehemently, to which I had no defense, because I was so unfamiliar with displays of love and affection. The triggering of his anxiety and my withdrawing was a constant minefield to negotiate.

WHAT I LEARNED

Things began to go off the rails as I began asserting my own needs and wants, such as taking time for myself to do my own hobbies. Before then, I would actually hide in the bathroom just so I could read a magazine in peace. Contrary to what it may sound like, Mark was not a tyrant, although early on it sometimes felt that way. He is truly a kind and gentle man, and an amazing father, but when we were younger, he was forceful in his demands of me, and I was a willing participant in placating his needs. What I didn't realize was that I was sacrificing my own. He was seeking reassurance due to his insecurities and anxieties, and it was my constant inability to state what was and was not okay (setting healthy boundaries) that haunted me.

This was the way our relationship played out for many years, and while my husband's obsessive tendencies relaxed a bit over time, and my communication skills improved, there was still precious little attention paid to my needs, even from myself, because my lack of awareness prevented it. It was a long road of discovery for me to find those linkages between what I experienced in the past and my current behaviors, and then to identify the emotional content of those memories to help me understand what actually was happening (my traumatic response being triggered) versus what I believed was happening (a "normal" relationship).

LEARNING TO FEEL

Once you have made those connections on your own between your memories and your behavior, you can see how you responded and what you learned from the internalization of it, which may not accurately reflect the event. Once you can recognize and accept that it is a mix of memories, perceptions, experiences and interpretations of those experiences that influenced you, you can begin to let go of the emotion attached to the event. But before you can do that, you need to actually allow yourself to feel the emotion that you've worked so hard to avoid, or simply blamed on your caregiver(s) or someone else, for their behavior.

Reacting to their behavior, even years later, is a start. Feeling some emotion in response to those circumstances is giving yourself permission to feel. Once I identified my trauma, I was angry about what I felt was betrayal, particularly from abandonment by my father. However, this opened the door for forgiveness, which facilitates healing. My father, and also my mother, passed away long before I was able to conceive of these things, let alone articulate them, so I had no avenue for closure with my parents except to forgive them. Ultimately, it is your responsibility to heal from this experience, because unfortunately, no one else can do it for you. No one else is you; therefore no one else can organize and assimilate the information that you have gathered in your consciousness and your body, in the form of memories, physical reactions and emotional responses, to learn to let go and finally heal.

Forgiveness is quite simply the only ability you have to take power back from that situation long ago. Although blame can genuinely be assigned to someone else, it is not helpful to point fingers for the sake of being right or being vindicated. Taking a neutral stance while seeing all of the contributing factors in your life, while acknowledging your responses and their accuracy, can help you understand and accept why these feelings are coming up, which is the precursor to sitting with emotions. To me, there is a difference between doing things that could re-traumatize you by reliving the past or triggering yourself by reexperiencing the emotions from your memories, and carefully creating conditions in a controlled manner/setting in which you feel the emotions as an adult, with the intention to discover, release and heal them.

Understand that it is okay to feel emotions that were absent at the time and to finally feel what you never allowed yourself to feel before. In the next exercise, practice sitting with emotions, identifying them, labeling them, feeling where sensations take place in the body, noticing what you do and how you respond when the feelings arise. These are all important steps in the process. You may want to revisit these steps many times, to "practice" letting the feelings happen, before moving on. When you can accept that you have an internalization or interpretation of the event that is only a memory based on old responses that no longer reflect reality, you are ready to assimilate this information into a larger picture of your life. Realizing that your personal power is dependent on not being enslaved by memories, emotions or debilitating thoughts and behaviors is the key to your freedom from trauma.

LEARNING TO HEAL

Before I delve into the hot topic of sitting with emotion, there are some other helpful self-healing exercises, such as recognizing and challenging negative self-talk, using affirmations and reframing victimhood. Recognizing and replacing negative self-talk is crucial because it forms your opinion of yourself. I was a menace to myself because I would scold myself mercilessly for any perceived errors I had made. I found fault with anything about myself, especially if it involved my appearance or level of competence, and discerned that to be the reason for my failures or my lack of importance. Thoughts sculpt your reality. Challenge those thoughts, and ask yourself whether they are really true.

Negative thoughts are self-sabotage, and countering them requires specific strategies. Alter them to a more realistic state-ment or, ideally, a positive thought that is truthful, which may be even more beneficial. Be specific. Instead of catastrophizing by say-ing, "I am such a failure at parenthood," say to yourself, "I could have handled my son's outburst better without yelling. I will try to count to ten before speaking next time, to gather my thoughts." Or say, "My son loves me and I love him. We will work out a better solution together, but it will start by me asking him what is really going on."

I had a hard time with affirmations, because they often sounded hokey to me, especially using "I" statements, such as "I am a worth-while person." I had to come up with mantras of my own that were relevant to my situation, more process oriented and more like mindfulness exercises. The ones that worked for me and got me through my most painful experiences were "The only way is through," "Expect nothing, accept everything," "Just put one foot in front of the other" and "This too shall pass." You can create affirmations or mantras, either in your mind (keep it limited in number and simple) or on paper (as many as you find helpful or effective) and put them up in your home, either on your fridge or taped to your computer screen so that you have to read them before you can flip the page over the screen to use it. If coming up with your own affirmations and mantras doesn't work for you, there is no shortage of affirmations and inspirational quotes to be found online. A quick Google search of "positive affirmations" should do the trick in finding one that resonates with you.

PREPARE YOUR SAFE SPACE

Sitting with emotion is probably the hardest part of the work you will do. This is the part that requires your courage, because virtually no one wants to revisit painful memories or experience the betrayals you never recognized as such. However, by going through with this, and allowing yourself to actually feel the emotions, you make way to surpass your trauma. After all, you need to feel the emotion to let it go. This requires a safe space.

A psychologist's office is usually considered a safe space, but perhaps it is not for you. For whatever reason, you have chosen to take on this task yourself to overcome your trauma, instead of consulting professional help. You will need to find a safe space though, which may be a physical space like a meditation room, whether it is at a facility like a community center, gym or possibly at home. Sometimes it can be hard to carve out time and physical space to make this happen. It may require using your garage, a home office or a spare bedroom so that you are not disturbed. Perhaps if you don't have this space, or you have a spouse or children who may interrupt you, you can use your living room, but wake up earlier or stay up later than everyone else so that you have dedicated quiet time and space for this practice.

You're going to hear that word a lot: *practice*. There are several practices employed in this journey, but it starts with finding a quiet, ideally private space where you can perform the previous exercises of remembering the events of the past and making connections to current circumstances, using your journal entries as prompts. The goal is to make the connections between your memories, so that the adult reactions you may now experience will inform you of the emotional responses that were missing for you as a child. The more private your space, the better.

SITTING WITH EMOTION

You may have difficulty experiencing emotional release. Emotional release is an adaptive strategy for coping, especially with things outside of your control (such as in your past), and is a healthy and effective way to manage stressful situations. If you have no reaction to your own most impactful memories, perhaps you can use other things that have stirred up emotion for you in the past. Is there a movie that is a tear-jerker that really gets to you? If so, can you think of a scene that somehow reminds you of your own situation, and perhaps that is the reason it affects you this way? How about music? Is there a specific song that gets to you? Another option is to think of a tragic story that really affected you, whether it was a news story or a situation involving someone you know. If it really hits home, then pay attention because that is something that you can use to kickstart your emotional release. If you can use these more automatic emotional reactions as a "head start" to begin the process, then you can reflect on your own memories after that point, using the momentum of the emotional release to keep it going.

Use your journal to revisit the memories and the connections you have made between your trauma and your current life circumstances. Once you are able to recognize the feelings arising in you, let them out! Allow the tears to flow, the rage to surface or whatever is happening to happen. If you need to scream into a pillow, or punch it, these are safe ways to express what you have been suppressing all along. If you have an empty chair handy, you can also say (out loud) what you always wanted to say to someone by picturing them in it, or you can journal about what you would like to say to someone. When I cried myself to sleep at night for months after my breakdown, I was letting out the pent-up emotions that were trapped in me for so long. Doing it this way felt like the safest option.

If you think that this may be too much for you right from the start, or if at any point you find this is too intense an exercise, you can always stop and go back to the breathing and grounding exercises. You can make another attempt using some memories that are less emotionally loaded, to ease into the process, before continuing on to try to dig up heavier emotions. For instance, is there a more recent memory that you can use? Something less intense, say a disappointment or an irritation. Did someone cut you off in traffic today? How did you react? With anger or frustration? How about failing an important test, say for employment? How did you react to that disappointment, that failure? Were you sad, or angry at yourself? Perhaps you can recall an argument with a friend or your partner? This is designed to be a less intense experience, but an emotional one nonetheless.

Instead of simply remembering it objectively as before, this time you want to revisit that moment, to reexperience that flaring of emotion. Now, sit with that feeling for at least a few moments and pay attention to it. Try to locate where it takes place in your body. Take note whether it was in the heart, the throat, the limbs, the stomach or wherever. Note this in your journal too, as it may come in handy later, when we look at embodiment. As previously mentioned, if at any time you begin to feel anxiety or an intense reaction, stop the exercise and use either the breathing or grounding exercise in Chapter 1 until you are calm and relaxed again.

When you realize that you have experienced adverse childhood experiences, it is a revelation, but an unwelcome one, because they have had such an enduring impact on your psyche and consequences for your life. It is not easy to integrate this into your life without feeling like a victim. Make no mistake: you are a victim of emotional neglect; however, to overcome this victim state, you must ultimately take responsibility for your healing and your life. Blaming is an attractive response to the trauma inflicted upon you, intentional or not, but it is by letting go of blame that you will be able to take the reins of your life and move it forward. Reframing victimhood involves taking personal responsibility, and challenges you to see yourself as the one in the driver's seat—therefore no longer seeing yourself as the victim. Both of these topics, plus the role of perspective, are dealt with in more detail in the next chapter.

4

Acceptance: How Do I Get Beyond This?

HOW TO MOVE forward—this is the million-dollar question, isn't it? There are a few tools you can use to tackle this topic, such as the roles of perspective, victimhood, forgiveness, gratitude and acceptance. Acknowledging the hurt that was caused by your care-givers is an important step before tackling the other tools though. You may feel angry, betrayed, cheated, despairing, broken-hearted or lost. You could feel a number of other emotions, or all of the above. The tools presented in this chapter helped me to overcome those feelings and move forward with my life. I hope they can do the same for you.

This chapter's lesson is for you to view your life differently. It is to remove or minimize the role of victimhood in your life and replace the story in your head that you may have about trauma, such as "It ruined my life." That means you must recognize your perspective as a potential source of misinformation. Forgiving yourself and others for their part in creating the trauma in your life is another area for examination. Gratitude and acceptance are even more potent tools for healing. This means that you need a new perspective in order to be able to help yourself. This requires a lot of openness and self-compassion: openness to see the circumstances of your life in a different light and self-compassion for the mistakes you may have made.

Naturally, we all make mistakes—this is how we learn. Accepting this can open us to the possibility of forgiveness. Forgiving those who disappointed, abused, neglected or betrayed us, whether intentionally or not, is an especially important act, but forgiving yourself (for any real or perceived mistakes, deficits or whatever else) is even more profound in this journey to enlightenment. This requires self-love and acceptance. The old adage "Time heals all wounds" is incomplete. Over time, you can learn to accept all that has happened to you, and it is acceptance that actually heals the wounds. Acceptance of the role you and your family played in your trauma relies heavily on a change in perspective.

PERSPECTIVE

Sometimes it is hard to get some distance and objectivity once you realize the harm that was done to you at an early age. Understandably, you may be struggling to deal with it, having recently come to the realization of the trauma you experienced as a child, and being overwhelmed by its impact on your life. Emotional neglect is virtually undetectable, by anyone, including you, because there are few observable symptoms, and those that are noticeable (withdrawn behavior, for example) don't automatically tend to be connected to trauma.

Emotional neglect robs you of your ability to discern what is right for you, prevents you from engaging meaningfully in the world and leaves you feeling a lack of love and belonging or any sense that you even matter. With no attention being paid to you, learning about intimacy is virtually impossible, and you are bereft of the ability to connect with people, creating serious repercussions in mental and emotional stability beginning in youth and bleeding well into adulthood. It can take the form of depression, anxiety, low or no self-worth, next to no social skills and problems forming or maintaining healthy relationships.

At a young age, your perspective of what is normal can become skewed because, being in the care of unskilled or lackadaisical care-givers, you have no other perspective from which to view the situation. Your "normal" really isn't normal, and it takes a lot to shift your perspective without an awareness of what love and support truly look like. It also takes a lot of healing work to undo the damage after realizing that what you thought was a normal life growing up was anything but. Without awareness, personal perspective is fixed, introspective and wholly influenced by your upbringing and society, by externally accepted values and other people's opinions.

Once you recognize that your perspective has the potential to be faulty or limited, it is easier to accept that trauma could be so pervasive in its hold over you. After all, I participated in "normal" activities, such as soccer and baseball, as a child and had friends. I was a decent student and never made trouble at school, mostly to stay out of the teacher's way though. I didn't trust adults and was basically afraid of them, so I avoided being seen by them to avoid "consequences." So, although I probably appeared like a regular kid, albeit a quiet one, I don't think anyone would have seen anything out of the ordinary in my behavior or assumed anything negative about my upbringing. I had everyone fooled, myself included.

Generally speaking, I don't think that parents consider their capacity for inflicting emotional harm on their children, and there-fore there is great potential and risk for serious damage being done to children when the parents themselves are unaware of their own trauma. When parents harm their children, they may be reenacting harms done to them or emotionally reacting to their life circum-stances, and while they are in that reactive state, they are taking it out on an easy, available target with little consideration of the con-sequences for the child. The sad fact is, parents are doing the best they can with the skills they have, and unfortunately some perform abysmally, while others are able to balance the joys, the challenges and the tedium of child-rearing more easily, particularly if they are not dealing with trauma themselves.

It would take a lot of openness and forgiveness to get beyond situations of violent abuse. However, trying to "take a walk in someone else's shoes" is the best way to build empathy. Seeing another's perspective gives you access to a bigger picture. It gives you some objectivity and allows you to detach from the struggles of your life (your subjective experience), making room for empathy to grow. While this may not always be possible, having some empathy for your parents can go a long way toward changing your perspective, as you attempt to understand them. Learning as much as you can about your parents and their own upbringing may help you to empathize with them. It can help you to understand their actions and their intentions a little better so that ultimately you can forgive them for their shortcomings and mistakes, in short, their humanity.

MY PERSPECTIVE CHANGE

At first, I kept wanting to blame my parents for "doing" something to me, but I couldn't put my finger on what, exactly, they "did." I just had this vague sense of injustice, and it explained why, as a teenager, I would sneak away to my room and flail wildly as I listened to my music, privately dancing away my pain. I had no understanding of why I felt that way at the time. So it finally made sense that when, as an adult, I looked back on my "It's not fair" memory (mentioned in Chapter 2) for the first time, I felt such a justified sense of betrayal, knowing that they hadn't provided for me emotionally. Placing blame was an attractive response in answer to all the questions I had about why I was the way I was, and to at least have *some* reason for why I turned out the way I did.

As I later realized, it was more accurately what my parents *didn't* do that was at fault. It was their frequent inattention, a lack of noticing my emotional needs and consequently not meeting them in any meaningful way, that left such a deep impact on my psyche. This resulted in me not feeling "seen," in me internalizing that I didn't matter, and it fostered a profound lack of self-worth. However, it was very cathartic to be able to feel anger, bitterness, *something*, after years of dissociation, numbed emotions and depression. It was short-lived, though, as the reaction felt hollow somehow. I knew beyond any doubt that they didn't mean for it to be this way.

I was some way down the path of healing at this point and, looking back, I realized that more was going on than simply having disinterested, indifferent or inept parents. I realized that I actually factored into this equation somewhere. My perspective, built by trauma, had distorted my interpretation of events and my world view. I thought I had uninvolved (true), unloving (untrue) parents. Once my eyes were opened to this new perspective, I began to see a bigger picture.

A pattern had evolved throughout my life, and it illuminated for me the source of my despair, my alone-ness and my subsequent descent into depression. I realized I had become depressed and withdrawn as a *result* of my upbringing, not simply that I was innately defective, or "born this way." I wasn't just a helpless creature, having no ability to effect change on my own life, as it had once seemed. This was quite a revelation for me. I had not only an explanatory source of my problems (my parents' lack of attunement to me and not attending to my needs) but also my habitual response to events (a generalized sense of worthlessness, being unlovable and invisible) that had become entrenched in my subconscious thoughts, my feelings about myself and subsequently my actions. I had to accept that I played a part in perpetuating my trauma, in part because of the circumstances, genetic makeup and temperament, even though it was truly not my fault.

I had to look for proof that my parents loved me so that I could move forward. Some things could not be accounted for by an explanation of unloving parents, such as the fact that they sent me on a Mediterranean educational cruise at the age of fourteen, which was probably the most formative experience of my life. I recognized that they actually *wanted* something good for me, rather than viewing it as I had previously, which I felt was like getting a "day pass" from a metaphorical jail whenever something good happened. I also guessed that there were experiences that affected their lives to lead them to parent in a particular way. I started to see them as people instead of aloof ogres, which was hard for me in my underdeveloped state, since I didn't really understand people in the first place. It was seeing their faults and flaws that gave me a broader perspective and a better understanding of humanity—theirs as well as my own.

Although things that happened to you may not be your own fault, and despite the fact that these things may have happened to you when you were a child, at a developmental stage where you were not equipped to deal with the struggle, pain or bewilderment of why this happened, it is still your burden and responsibility as an adult to learn how to heal from these experiences. By seeing yourself as the prime mover of your life, you take your power back from your childhood experience, and get out from under your parental influences and childhood conditioning. You go from being the victim to being the victor. This is the lesson that maturity teaches us. By viewing your life as your own, you actually own it! You own your experience and can see trauma as being part of your life story, rather than a tragedy that stopped you from living. This is a way to integrate your trauma into your life by accepting it and assimilating the lessons from it into your thoughts, which will affect your actions and feelings.

Perspective can also change very suddenly when an unexpected event happens, such as a car crash, the death of a loved one or—

ahem—an emotional breakdown. The insight may not come right away, or it may not come at all, if you sweep it under the rug, preferring to avoid the resulting pain by burying your head in the proverbial sand, and to avoid the eventual aftermath. Ignoring the problem won't make it go away in any arena of life. In fact, the more you ignore symptoms or avoid the difficulties in dealing with the problem, the more prolonged the duration of the problem, the deeper the impact and the more profound the pain will be with the inevitable reckoning.

It is better to use the tools of your insight, gained as they were through experience, however unpleasant, and equipping you with a perspective that would have remained unseen had it not been for this thing that happened to you. Insight is a powerful tool for understanding yourself and others, and a great motivator for change, especially if you realize that something has been holding you back and you no longer are willing to accept this situation and wait for the circumstances to change on their own.

Once you realize that the path you were on was always part of the trajectory of your own unique individual experience, whether you asked for that experience or not, you can take full responsibility for your life, which frees you from the imprisonment of victimhood. No experience is going to be the same for anyone, so endlessly comparing yourself to others is a waste of time and energy. While some people may seem to have it easier, I'm sure we can all agree that life isn't easy for anyone. Why not make it easier for yourself? You can choose a new perspective as quickly as you can change your mind, but to do this, you must have full acceptance of all that has gone on before. You are literally changing from a fixed mindset to one of growth. Why not focus on what unites us as human beings instead of focusing on the false assumptions and useless agonizing of comparing yourself to others? As the saying goes, comparison is the thief of joy.

Gaining new insights through a change in perspective and building empathy is what will help you in connecting with others, which encourages having mutually supportive relationships. Having empathy is the building block for love. Learning to love and trust were my big barriers to happiness and wholeness. I didn't realize it was a debilitating lack of trust that was preventing me from having the relationship I truly wanted, and it took me a long time to identify that trust was the issue at the heart of my trauma. This insight illuminated the whole reason for my failure to connect with Myles and was the start of my learning in earnest.

Perspective Exercise

Think about what perspective you could change that would make your life easier. Use your journal, and write down a key area in your life that is holding you back. Try to think of the issue from all sides. Take the perspective of your best friend, for example. How would this person describe your situation? Would this match your perspective? If not, why the discrepancy? Really examine it. Is there more than one way to view the situation? Is there a way that you can reframe it to understand it or relate to it better when viewed differently? Is it possible that there is a more objectively realistic perspective? If you can, talk to your friend about your situation and get their perspective. Seeing a different perspective can give you valuable new information and understanding, especially of others. Gaining insight through a perspective shift can illuminate the path toward better relationships, because in order to love others in a healthy way, you must first have empathy, which requires said perspective.

As I have mentioned, this is a practice, and something you will likely return to again and again. I found that having a new perspective makes doing the exercises much more manageable, which in turn makes the process more achievable.

FORGIVENESS

Once the emotional content of these traumatic experiences—or at least, your reaction to them, and the power it wields over you—is lessened, it is easier to learn forgiveness. Forgiveness can take different forms. Certainly, the most obvious way is learning to forgive those who have emotionally injured you in your childhood. You may also find it necessary to learn forgiveness of yourself, whether you blame yourself for the traumatic events or you still feel shame for disappointing parents, not getting parental approval or being made to feel not worthwhile. Lack of self-worth is a particularly damaging effect of trauma, and forgiveness of self can help you to understand that you were a child, with no ability to better handle your childhood situation. Having a traumatic response to caregiver neglect is a completely understandable reaction.

Forgiveness is an act that is more beneficial to the forgiver than to the forgiven. It is an act of acceptance of the facts surrounding what happened to you, and a letting go of the emotional grip that it has over you. Forgiveness of others can be difficult, especially in the face of overt physical, verbal or emotional abuse, which are intentional acts, whatever the intent of the abuser and however damaged they themselves are. As an adult, you might eventually be able to get past the anger and betrayal to acknowledge that your caregivers may have done the best that they could with what little skills they had (if you're a saint!), but it still comes down to forgiveness being about you rather than the perpetrator(s). Forgiveness is a release of the hold that others have over you. You are releasing the power they have over you so that you can claim it for yourself. This is the purpose of forgiveness, and the process allows you to reconcile what happened to you with how you want to live your life going forward.

Forgiveness Exercise

Try this simple forgiveness exercise. Use a piece of paper, your journal or your smartphone to record two lists of people in your life: those who supported you and those who did not. If one person supported you in one way and not another, put them on both lists. Go down the list and name those who did out loud, by saying, "Thank you, _____." To those who didn't, say, "I forgive you, _____." By doing this, you recognize your supporters, while also releasing the energy trapped inside you in response to your abusers or detractors. The end goal is integration of your life events into a conception of life that includes and accepts all of your experiences, in order to have a holistic view of it and a healthier outlook on life. To end the interminable, fruitless search for happiness is to accept your life as it is, in full knowledge of the power you have to change it.

Forgiveness of yourself is equally important, and sometimes even more difficult than forgiving someone else. When dealing with shame and lack of self-worth due to neglect, we as children may have internalized that we were "bad" and deserved poor treatment, or that what we "did" was unforgivable, such as not living up to our parents' supposed or real expectations. These things get trapped inside of us, lingering within us for decades. This is why self-compassion is important. Remembering that you were a child in circumstances out of your control can help you empathize with the child you once were. Ask yourself how would you have been able to change your circumstances? Answer: you couldn't. Remind yourself that as a child, you had no control over how you were raised or the experiences you had to endure. It wasn't your fault, and forgiving yourself, even if only for not being able to detect this earlier, especially if you have had lifelong lack of self-love and self-worth, is a very therapeutic thing that you can do for yourself.

GRATITUDE

Once you forgive the people and aspects of life that contributed to your traumatic experience, you can use another tool: gratitude. Gratitude has such enormous power. Although it may be extremely difficult to see how anyone could be grateful for such awful experiences as neglect or abuse, this perspective can be achieved if you so choose. This isn't the best approach for everyone; however, you *can* be grateful for getting through and surviving such circumstances, if not being grateful for the event itself. Some may be able to integrate their traumatic experience through forgiveness. If you are able to move past the emotional triggers of your family relationships and have gratitude for the perspective you have gained, that is terrific. If you would rather leave family dynamics behind and focus on your journey, your resolve and your desire to live life to the fullest, that is equally fantastic.

There is no one-and-only method to surpass your trauma, but the steps outlined in this book are concrete actions you can take, however insignificant they may seem, to create change in your life and create ease in your body, mind and soul. Small actions add up over time, and this is what changes habits, even if they are habits formed from trauma. You can't be in gratitude and be resentful at the same time, so find something to be grateful for every day, and see if you can extend it to the circumstances of your trauma. It is an exercise in repetition, which has powerful effects on your mindset and in your heart-space, the seat of emotions.

Gratitude is a powerful practice to alter your thoughts. It forces you to really notice and appreciate what you have. Use it in combination when you recognize that you are engaging in negative self-talk by immediately switching to finding gratitude for something. Gratitude can short-circuit negative self-talk and will begin to alter your perceptions of what is true by getting you to focus on what you have, not what you think you lack. When you have gratitude, you come to appreciate even the smallest things that you have, even if it's just a favorite pair of shoes, or that one person in your life you are comfortable talking to. Gratitude can alter your mindset and the way your brain perceives information by replacing an automatic negative slant with a more positive outlook. When you realize what you have, you recognize that something has been provided to you, or someone in your life values you, even if that person is yourself. Something inside you has given you that strength, resilience or ability to cope and survive, and if that only came from within, and if you survived with virtually no supports whatsoever, then you are indeed a powerhouse!

Gratitude is an act of mindfulness. It alters your thoughts by attaching them to a positive emotion, which creates a positive feedback loop in your brain. It actually trains your brain for happiness. But you need to practice. I defaulted to it whenever I went down a familiar path of self-pity, self-loathing or just hating my life. I began appreciating. I even became grateful for all of the painful experiences of the past, for all of the lessons it taught me. I had to practice and practice for months and months. It didn't happen all at once, and it was non-linear. The pain would come in waves, contracting me emotionally at the hardest moments of denial and then expanding when I felt a sense of calm acceptance, until I felt only the acceptance.

Then one day, I stopped feeling the pain and suffering. This wasn't a case of me convincing myself of something that wasn't true or denying the pain. Believe me, losing the love of my life was no picnic. I felt an enormous hole in my life and had difficulty picturing a future without him. What I finally realized from the experience was that I was a whole person already, needing no other person to complete me—neither Myles nor Mark—not even my parents. The happiness borne of contentment was already mine. It provided me so much peace of mind, which was ultimately what was missing in my life's journey. It's amazing how something so simple works so well. Gratitude is a game-changer in the context of trauma, because it changes your perspective, giving you a more accurate, nuanced and mature view of the world.

Gratitude Exercise

Try this basic gratitude exercise. Make a list of all the things and people for which you are grateful. When you find yourself descending into a depressive state or punishing yourself with negative self-talk, stop (I think of a stop sign in my mind) and remind yourself of that for which you are grateful. Using gratitude to surmount your trauma is the act of you literally changing your mind (or your brain, really).

Much of the message in this book is that the work requires practice and repetition. Things like forgiveness, gratitude, replacing negative self-talk with self-love and acceptance all require repetition because repetition is how it integrates into your consciousness. It is by repetition that we learn because we learn by reinforcement. That is why when you study, you reread and rewrite your work. Studying is just like practice. You study to learn new things and integrate them into your knowledge. You practice to learn new skills by applying the concepts you have learned and to alter your behaviors into new patterns. Repetition ... it works. Practice forgiveness, repeat, practice gratitude, repeat, practice self-compassion, repeat, practice self-love, repeat, practice acceptance, repeat.

Once you have accepted, and perhaps even have gratitude for your experience, or at least for what you have learned, you can then begin to deal with other aspects of experience and begin other work. Learning to self-soothe, for instance, is an important developmental milestone to achieve. You build emotional self-reliance so that you can trust yourself to get through this process by connecting to your authentic self, the truest and innermost essence of you. However, learning acceptance is what will fully empower you. It is where personal power is derived. The next step in achieving this is the work of reparenting and inner child work.

5

Reality Check:
Can I Handle the Truth?

ONCE A SHIFT in perspective occurs for you, other issues and experiences may rear their ugly heads. You may experience denial from this new perspective, about how your life has been affected by trauma, such as being held back in life and kept from pursuing your passions and fulfilling relationships. Perhaps now you recognize that your needs have changed in ways you are unwilling to accept at this point, such as getting out of a dysfunctional or unsatisfying relationship. Your world view, originally based out of trauma, may now be challenged or altered, and it requires work from you to adapt to this new perspective of the world. It may challenge your old view of things, which no longer fits in your life or serves your needs.

You may now understand that your ideas about the world, which you adopted from your parents, may be wrong or may have become fixed by a mindset of scarcity. You may come to realize that there is an alternative to the toxic relationships you've experienced. There may be denial about where your old life guided you, and disappointment about what might have been if your life had turned out differently. There may be grief for the life you are going to lose or, even more devastating, the one you never had. This can devolve into purposelessness, because it may feel like life has passed you by or been a waste up until the realization that this trauma took place or took such a toll on your life.

The truth is that life probably turned out a lot differently than you had expected or hoped. As I explained in the previous chapter, taking a new perspective of your life can help tremendously. It can ease the transition from your denial of what your life actually has been, as opposed to what you thought it was supposed to be, to now realizing what it could have been and accepting all that has come to pass. Techniques like inner-child work, reparenting and embodiment practices can help soften the blow and promote healing through learning to let go of disappointments, resentments or rage that may be trapped in the body. Learning to accept what you may have missed out on growing up can help you avoid becoming a victim of circumstance. You also learn to manage your own emotional state instead of looking for an external source of comfort (like another person) to do the emotional work for you. It was a combination of these techniques, in addition to my shift in perspective, that allowed me to check in with the reality of my life and better handle the truth of it.

SELF-SOOTHING

Learning self-soothing as a child is one of the major milestones of development. It is a move away from a stage when the child is dependent on caregivers to soothe them when they are in distress to a stage of more self-reliance. When a child gets hurt and needs someone to wipe away the tears and provide comfort, the parent or caregiver who provides this models soothing behaviors to the child so that he or she can eventually learn to regulate emotions on his or her own.

When a parent does not provide this soothing, it leaves the child to seek soothing through external sources (other people and/or things), therefore skipping the self-soothing milestone altogether. Even the comfort of a stuffed animal is not sufficient if you haven't had any modeling of soothing behavior. If you constantly lean on people to seek reassurance or frequently rely on substances to relax instead of drawing on your own resources to calm yourself and resolve your anxiety, you may be substituting these habits for the self-soothing that you never learned in childhood. Trauma can result from the neglect of caregivers to attend to you in times of distress. Left unchecked and unaddressed over time, it can result in maladaptive coping behaviors such as hypervigilance, numbing, codependency, self-harm, substance abuse and other addictive behaviors or disorders.

Perhaps you can identify with some of these issues. I know I can. Not learning self-soothing is like not knowing the next steps in a dance: it stops you in your tracks. Self-soothing is the beginning of learning to stand on your own two feet and supporting yourself, physically, mentally and emotionally. Learning to calm yourself and being your own source of soothing as an adult, especially in the absence of family support, is one of the best things you can do for your psyche. It is the essence of maturity because you take control and responsibility for your thoughts, feelings and actions. It requires practice, because you may never have learned it growing up.

Self-soothing was the nexus of my inner-child work. I was introduced to inner-child work in a class, by finding or remembering a picture of myself as a four- or five-year-old child (I remembered a particularly forlorn-looking one of me), and whenever I engaged in negative self-talk, I was to imagine telling the child in that picture the same thing. Having two young children around that same age definitely helped me to effectively curb my negative self-talk, as it wasn't much of an imaginary leap to think of speaking to my own children in that way, which would have been completely unacceptable.

Negative self-talk skews your self-concept by convincing your-self of something that is not based in reality. Using acts of imagina-tion like in the previous example is a powerful way to counter that tendency. For example, I imagined my inner child to be my knight in shining armor, who had tirelessly protected me from further harm, even though her protection came with a price: keeping others at arm's length. However, I used this imagery to remind myself of how strong I actually was.

Acknowledging that there can be an alternative positive story about yourself is a great way to help bring awareness about how you have adopted particular thought patterns and adapted certain behaviors to fit the beliefs you had about yourself. By imagining yourself now as the hero, or perhaps even remembering who you once were, you can use this imagery as a source of comfort to rely on in times of distress instead of using other people or substances to prop you up. Integrating that person or persona into the land-scape of your mind is one way to help train you to self-soothe.

You can take other approaches to self-soothing as well, such as positive affirmations and self-care rituals. For me, a physical approach combined with my imagination worked best. In my most painful moments, I had to actually lie on the sofa and embrace myself while reminding myself that the little girl in me was doing her utmost to protect me from harm, rather than being at war with me. I imagined my valiant knight, in a fearsome suit of impenetra-ble black armor with blade-like protrusions that reminded me of feathers and a razor-sharp spear (my *Game of Thrones* influence is perhaps showing here). She watched over me, ever-present and ever-vigilant, for all the years of my life. I praised my inner child for her tireless, unyielding protection, metaphorically embracing her as I physically embraced myself. As I thanked her for her unwaver-ing dedication, I also told her that she had done her job well, and that her watch was finally over. It was time to rest. I said all of this in order to show myself the comfort, acceptance and love that I needed but was not provided to me, and that I could now provide for myself.

Inner Child Exercise

Imagine your own inner child, perhaps one you remember being as a child or one of your imagination. What does she or he look like? Do you want to imagine them as a heroic figure like mine, or think of how you remember yourself at a particular age, perhaps when you were most happy? Perhaps there is some other picture in your mind, like a superhero that you always wanted to be. Keep a clear picture or at least a good idea of what this person looks like in your mind's eye. Praise this child for their service to you, or remember being that happy child—what it actually felt like—and really let that sink in. If this is not something that works for you, try something different. For example, look in the mirror, then thank yourself, out loud, for your strength and courage in taking this journey. You may find when you are face to face with yourself, that it is easier to talk to you than to others.

That was always the case with me. I came up with a phrase that represented the essence of my learning. By distilling what I had recently learned into one succinct statement, I kept the message simple and easy to remember, with the aforementioned mantras like "Expect nothing, accept everything," "Just put one foot in front of the other" and so on. Sometimes I would talk to myself seriously, like I was revealing to my best friend an intimate secret or a very astute observation I had made. Talking to myself was easier than talking to someone else, because I was largely a loner who was much more comfortable with my own company. Talking to yourself works well if you are of a similar temperament, or if you are just trying to work this out on your own. Try coming up with ideas of your own if you prefer, until you find something that feels right. Go ahead: use your imagination, but keep it positive in terms of self-talk, focused on the young version of yourself, and how that child reacted to circumstances outside of his or her control.

REPARENTING

Reparenting encompasses learning to "pick yourself up and dust yourself off" when you have fallen down, so to speak, and to encourage yourself to carry on in the face of adversity. It sounds a lot like self-soothing, which is a childhood developmental milestone that you have had to relearn, but reparenting is more of an adult skill that builds on self-soothing. Self-soothing is a subjective experience where you are learning to internally comfort and calm yourself. With reparenting, you come at it from a more objective, "parental" perspective. You are literally taking on the role that your parents relinquished (perhaps unintentionally), in order to help you heal your inner child in adulthood and move your life forward.

Reparenting involves encouraging yourself, which promotes resilience, so that you begin to believe in your ability to take on further challenges. It paves the way for you to be able to identify who you are, what your values are (covered in the next chapter) and to uncover and subsequently to handle the emotional impact of your past in order to be your own emotional support. It is a lot to ask of yourself. Relying on people close to you for support is a normal part of being human. When you are denied this support in childhood, you are placed in a position of becoming that support for yourself as an adult in order to facilitate your own healing.

It takes a certain level of mental and emotional fortitude to be your own parental figure, and to take it on with no example set for you, but learning to be your own support first and foremost is of the utmost importance in order to heal yourself. If there are good examples for you to follow (aunts, uncles, grandparents), you could ask for support from these people too by talking with them. Your healing doesn't have to be a solo endeavor. The bulk of the burden, however, lies on you to make sense of your history while putting into practice the many strategies, exercises (physical, mental and emotional), thought-pattern changes and behavior modifications.

Reparenting also involves asserting that you are "enough" and have a right to be in the world. Self-worth is usually derived from the loving guidance, the care and the scaffold of support from your parents or caregivers, that teaches you that you have inherent value by virtue of being yourself. When parents are unable to give this type of support, you are tasked with providing yourself with this encouragement, belief and support. You come to understand and believe that you are just as worthy of love as anyone else, and you equally deserve a place in the world.

Admittedly, sufferers of trauma have hard lessons to learn, partly because we were never taught how to deal with life's ups and downs, and partly because the overall effect of emotional neglect leaves us impotent to deal with emotions because they have been so long repressed due to the love denied to us or the conditioning we received. Without emotions to guide us, our decision-making can be fraught with stress or rendered completely impossible. Decisions may be based on someone else's idea of what is appropriate, or rigid, brittle ideas you have developed of what you think is right based on others' opinions, with no inner knowing, because of a lack of identity or sense of selfhood to come to your own conclusions.

I remember one time when my parents took me to McDonald's and asked me what I wanted to order. I felt acute stress and anxiety from not knowing what to choose, without someone telling me what to do. I finally made a decision out of sheer panic, rather than out of choice, because I didn't realize that I actually had a choice. This mundane example shows how you can be suffering with something with no one being the wiser.

Reparenting gives you the ability to provide for yourself the care and attention you lacked as a child and, in the process, develop your own sense of self. Think of the positive attributes of a caregiver, and then try to be those things for yourself. For me, it mostly took the form of encouragement. I became my own cheerleader and my own champion. I picked what I believed to be my most admirable attribute—courage—and reminded myself often of the courage it took to do this work, to keep moving forward. I encouraged myself to carry on, which was very hard in my darkest hours.

I also prepared to defend myself, because I was doing things that I felt were necessary for me to experience, learn and heal. If anyone took offense to my process, I was not afraid to defend my position. I leaned on people as well, which was near impossible for me as a kid. I always thought I was on my own. But I asked for help (from my ex-husband, my sister, my brother-in-law and friends) and was surprised by how people went out of their way to help me. Didn't expect that! So, please, use your supports and get help from those you trust. However, do not doubt that your biggest support needs to be you. You must be able to help yourself first. Be your own hero. And as always, practice, practice, practice.

EMBODIMENT PRACTICES

The exercises in Chapter 3 had you practicing sitting with the emotions that arose as a result of your memory retrieval exercises. Embodiment is the gateway to allowing yourself to physically feel your body, so that the emotions are encouraged to come forth and reveal themselves to you. You can then integrate them into your experience, by first allowing yourself to feel them, then accepting them and the events that happened to you. Finally, you can transform them from trauma experiences into life experiences. By reframing your thinking, you can include what was once a traumatic experience as an objective event in your life. Dealing with the resulting emotions by addressing the trauma and accepting it is integration. Embodiment is the key to opening up your psyche through releasing trapped energy in the body from trauma, and it works in combination with all the other exercises previously mentioned to free you of emotional blockages by simply getting physical in a variety of ways.

Body awareness is generated by embodiment practices, which can include things like cardiovascular exercise or sports, and physical activities such as dance, martial arts and yoga. Each has its own merits and advantages. You may not like physical activity, but you won't have to be relegated to the gym in order to achieve body awareness. Some embodied activities could be considered recreation, such as hand-drumming, Tai Chi or Qigong. You can also practice self-touch, which is not as unseemly as it sounds.

Self-touch literally gets you in touch with your body, by taking your hands and placing them purposefully and intentionally upon different areas of your body so that you can recognize that area and familiarize yourself with your physicality. It seems very basic, but that is the point. You must start simple when unfamiliar or uncomfortable with yourself, because it is the basis of somatic healing, or body-based healing.

You can use cardiovascular exercise or weight training as one way to get familiar with your body, if you focus on the feeling in your muscles as they work (always using proper form!) and the air entering and being expelled from your lungs. However, be careful if it is in a gym, as the distractions may not allow for proper focus.

I found yoga to be one of the two most effective embodiment practices for me because I was stretching and really noticing my muscles, while focusing on my breath and learning acute body awareness by making small adjustments to my posture while in poses in order to have proper alignment. I really had to focus on proper form because the yoga teacher would sometimes even gently correct my body by putting her hands on me (with consent) to guide me to the proper postural alignment.

I found that the yogic teachings offered by the instructor confer benefits through its wisdom as well. Both the guidance and being in physical alignment made me feel so *peaceful*. Dance, however, was my favorite embodiment practice, and to me, it was not just recreation. It is one of my most enduring passions. I really let go when I dance. Ecstatic dance was particularly cathartic for me because it is so expressive. These activities are all fantastic ways to get in touch with your body, but self-touch is a more subtle, simple approach.

EMBODIMENT IN TRAUMA

Sometimes, trauma can lead you to cut yourself off from your body, as another layer of protection, as another way of numbing, in an attempt to defend against the hurt and suppress the invisible, soul-crushing vacuum of neglect. Your inner child may forever try to hold back the despair and emptiness that awaits you if you allow yourself to feel anything at all, starting with your physical self. Denying your physicality is an extension of denying your emotional pain, so the body is another avenue to that hurt. It is vitally important to treat the body as well as the mind in healing childhood trauma.

In my case, it was my physicality that saved me. I did many things over the years that kept my body engaged that were key to my discovery of self. For example, I participated in baseball, soccer, dancing, running, weight training, cycling, and later on, yoga, parkour, belly dancing and ecstatic dancing. As I previously mentioned, sex in particular was one of the only needs I managed to get met while I was married. After my divorce, I let my interests guide me, and these activities are what began to open me up. I was going out dancing with my friends, pursuing one of my greatest passions, and getting fulfillment and social interaction from that, as well as the benefits of embodied expression.

I also had a few experiences of intense physical and emotional release during my ecstatic dance sessions. I was able to make the connection that I would not have had that emotional release and the simultaneous "letting go" of contracted muscles, tissues and fibers, without that *expressive* physical activity. This gave me the insight that what I did physically actually mattered, particularly in my practice of ecstatic dance. I was able to conceptualize then that the overall effect that trauma has is this: the body remembers. Every emotional injury is like a body blow. Some wounds heal while others fester and grow until addressed and released, or in my case, they explode when something (or someone) comes along and rips open the ancient wound afresh.

AVOIDING RISK

My awareness was just in its initial stages when I met The One. Myles was my trigger, which is why I reacted so strongly to him. I had never wanted something, or someone, so much in my life. He was the dream I never knew I had. He was the literal embodiment (pun fully intended) of all my interests, preferences, passions and desires, even subconscious ones. Something about his particular energy tapped into my intuition to tell me that THIS experience was the path to my emancipation and living my best life, which is why I was so obsessed with him. However, my inner child (or the manifestation of my unconscious fears) was putting up walls, raising the drawbridge and getting ready for battle. No way was she going to let someone in again who could hurt me so deeply.

This made it so that I was unable to connect with Myles, at least not verbally. We had limited opportunities to talk already since he was a musician in the band that my friends and I would often see at the nightclub where we went dancing. We communicated mostly through glances or longing gazes, but that connection can only get you so far. We were both very nervous, although we could tell that we very much wanted to connect. After all, you don't carry on for two years awkwardly trying to talk to each other without any real feelings being there. I knew I was in love, and I know he was too. In lieu of speaking, we had a very unconventional way of communicating, by letting the lyrics of the music speak for us and indicate how we were feeling as we gazed at each other intensely. It was very romantic and very powerful. We were emotionally in tune, just not verbally, and it kept me from being able to meaningfully and practically engage with him in pursuing the most powerful feeling of love I have ever experienced.

I just wasn't far enough along in the process of learning about myself and my trauma when Myles rejected me soundly and conclusively, using the music to communicate to me that he didn't love me anymore, a moment for which I was wholly unprepared (and which happened on the eve of COVID lockdowns). The reason my life exploded into chaos was not only from my discovery of trauma, or even falling in love with someone who rejected me. It was that in the two years that I knew him, I constantly wrestled with the opposing forces of the pursuit of my heart's desire and the frustration of my traumatic response, which constantly stymied me and was a mystery to me at the same time. I was so impatient to learn all that I had missed, or had been delayed in learning, that I was being careless. I pursued him fearlessly and foolishly, without knowing where my blind spots were, and my naivete about feeling that this was "meant to be" put me at risk for emotional devastation. After having such a powerful reaction to him, I allowed myself to be vulnerable and invest my emotions fully before really getting to know him, which was my undoing.

I was only coming to the realization of my trauma about a month before my interactions with Myles came to an abrupt halt, which sent me into a spiral of pain, sorrow, denial and a prolonged dissociation that was extremely destructive in my life. The constant activation of my fight or flight response wore my body and nervous system down so that when the inevitable rejection (which I saw coming) arrived, the re-traumatization (which I could not foresee) was catastrophic. It was at this point that my inner child took over, wreaking havoc on my life. I took financial risks in an effort to regain control of my life, and to try to have something good happen, while distracting myself from the pain, since I had unintentionally (obviously!) re-traumatized myself.

TAKE YOUR TIME

It is very difficult to be aware of something when the scars that it leaves are the result of its absence rather than its presence. Emotional neglect created a massive blockage in me and set me up for a chaotic storm of emotional release, with significant collateral damage. I had only just begun my true and proper somatic healing practice, so I hadn't had the time to integrate why I was reacting to Myles in that way. Plus, there was a lot I didn't yet know about my social and emotional learning. I had to heal all of my wounds and deal with all of my issues in quick succession, which is why it was so incredibly painful. This is why a slower approach is best. Taking your time will pay off so that you have time to integrate the emotional impact of your past, while exploring your triggers, your emotional landscape and your physical being while keeping yourself safe from re-traumatization. You can use embodiment practices to help you gently encourage the release of emotions.

Self-Touch Exercise

To learn what self-touch is, try this: Sit in a chair with hands on your lap. Take your right hand and hold the crook of your left elbow. Notice the feeling of your hand on your arm, where they are connected. Feel the warmth of your hand and make note of the quality of the feeling of your arm being held. Close your eyes if it helps you focus on the sensation. Is your arm being fully supported and comfortable? Is the grip firm or soft? Can you feel where each individual finger is placed on your arm? Then, notice what your hand is feeling. Is it skin or fabric? If it is skin, notice the feeling of the skin of your hand on your arm. Is it warm? Do you feel hair? If it is fabric, is it

soft, fuzzy, stiff or scratchy? Notice the difference. There is a dis-
tinction between the feeling of your arm as it is being touched and
the feeling of your hand as it touches your arm. Next, take your left
arm and touch your right shoulder, making note of the same sensations as before from the two differing sensations of each body
part. If you are comfortable enough to continue, you can continue
touching various parts of your body, to get used to the sensation
of touch, with a very focused purpose, in a very intentional act of
self-awareness and perhaps even appreciation.

Remember what your arms, legs, shoulders, hands, feet, back
and so on do for you on a daily basis, carrying you from place to
place and lifting things. We often take these things for granted, but
it's actually pretty amazing how quickly our bodies respond to our
command. You can move on to your legs and then to parts of your
torso, and work toward the neck, head and face. Spend some more
time on the parts of your face, your ears, temples, top of your head,
back of your neck and so on. Touch each area specifically, perhaps
caressing or massaging yourself gently to acknowledge an appreciation for your physical being. Do this with as little distraction as
possible. Getting comfortable touching your own body has the same
effect as getting comfortable with your personality or your sense
of humor. You come to appreciate and be completely comfortable
with all aspects of who you are.

The purpose of this is to sensitize yourself to your physical
being, to make yourself aware of your sensations and, ultimately,
to make yourself aware of where you are holding your trauma so
that you can release it. Once you are used to this exercise, you can
alter it to include describing, out loud, what it is that you feel. For
example, is your arm soft? Hairy? Muscular? Say it out loud so that
you can learn to accept yourself for who and what you are, without
judgment. After practicing this, if you can, move on to pairing the
exercise with affirmations or compliments about yourself, such as,
"I like my shoulders." Do and say what works for you. Pay attention
to what your body is telling you as well. If you notice aches or pains

that aren't due to any obvious cause and weren't there before, this may be an area to focus on to release that energetic block.

This is an introduction to body awareness that, in combination with the other exercises I have presented in previous chapters, can help you to make those connections to what traumatized you in the past and work to release that pain. Once you have taken on these practices more regularly and are starting to be accepting of yourself, physically and emotionally, it can create a sense of hope that you can change your life.

6

Hope: Can I Create a New Life for Myself?

CREATING A NEW life for yourself may seem like a pretty lofty goal, I imagine. I want to assure you that despite the lack of awareness that defined and shaped your past, it is possible. After working through the exercises in the preceding chapters and building some confidence in the idea of getting through all the emotional turmoil of the past, you broaden your capacity to let new ideas form in your mind and to make way for new, previously inconceivable ones. Trauma can narrow your thinking and limit your experience. Minimizing the effects of the stress response of the brain to the autonomic nervous system, using the exercises, encourages changes in your psyche from self-doubt to self-knowledge, from fear to trust in yourself and a sense of control over your life. The path is now laid before you to conceive of such things as a new job opportunity or a new relationship to unfold in your life. These are the things that create hope.

When changes begin to take shape, you dare to dream a bit bigger and to believe that you can do the things or have what it is that you want in your life. Determining what is important to you and what you want in your life directly reflects your values. To create change in your life, you'll likely need to adjust your goals. Your goals are reflections of what you value, what you want to spend your time on and with whom you want to spend it. Identity is the basis for your values because it is your definition of self. Without identity, your own values cannot form. Before I talk too much about values, though, I will address the foundational aspect of identity.

IDENTITY

Identity initially originates from parental or caregiver influences, but generally changes as you mature. Initially it can derive from other people in your life and sometimes activities as well, until you have learned to define it for yourself. Remember that "what you do" is not all that you are, any more than your name, skin color or body shape defines who you are. You are not what other people think you are or expect you to be, either. You are a complex combination of experiences and behaviors with an individual temperament that is unique. Instead of asking yourself *Who am I?*, start with *What do I want?* What you want is a much easier topic to tackle, and it gives you a far better indication of where you should put your focus than the indistinct and philosophical *Who am I?*, yet you can sometimes continue to grapple with ongoing identity issues with a backdrop of childhood trauma.

Identity defines who you are as a whole person in all aspects of your life. It can be subtly or overtly influenced by the people in your circle and by family in particular. If you find that you act in differing ways around different people, you can relax because this is normal. We often tailor our behavior to different people and situations because in society, it is natural to want to belong to the group, and adjusting to match someone's mood or mirroring other people's behavior is often a quick way to do this. Group dynamics, however, are not to be confused with identity. Identity is your internal compass. It is a sense of yourself and should ideally only be determined by you.

However, if you act against your own inner knowledge of what you want to do, or contrary to how you think or feel, especially to please others, beware. You may be acting out of habit to fulfill the demands of others, like an externally influenced form of the so-called autopilot, rather than acting on your own desires or according to your true nature. This habitual response is conditioned, reinforced from acceptance by your caregivers and peers, and then repeated by you because of that acceptance. Therefore, an identity is usually passed down to you from the interactions with your parents. Sometimes, though, it is thrust upon you.

The position of family may be of paramount importance in your family of origin. Your ethnic background may be the primary focus. You may be told what religion to practice. Even your recreation preferences may be prescribed to you, such as sports, art or music. You may carry on in these activities as an adult, but ultimately you must decide whether they actually have meaning for you or not. Don't get me wrong. I'm not knocking all those years of piano lessons or hockey practice. These things provide tangible benefits in learning and have likely shaped you in positive ways that you may not have thought about. They may even have introduced you to important people in your life. However, that doesn't mean these things can't be examined and reevaluated. Taking stock of what—and who—is present in your life is a worthy exercise, particularly if there are aspects of your life that aren't working for you.

It is well within your power to direct your life independently, and to decide whether or not to include people. Parting ways with those whom you have long known (or always known), is hard, but having the insight, skill and nerve to do so comes down to a few things: experience, understanding and knowing oneself. Experience shows you what you can expect from the other person, understanding tells you not to have preconceived ideas of the outcome of the situation, but knowledge of oneself is the most important because you know instinctively whether or not you want to try repairing the relationship. I'm certainly not suggesting that you go off and flippantly dump your friends or family after a falling out and run off blindly and recklessly to go "find yourself." You may quickly find yourself pretty lonely if you make rash decisions to end your relationships without due consideration.

Working to repair relationships is preferable because having a cohesive support group to love and understand you is what keeps you stable and feeling supported. Doing this is what makes relationships strong and what keeps us happy. When people are a support, you want to keep them in your life. Some relationships, however, make us unhappy or create inordinate distress. You have to figure out whether someone is toxic for you, because the danger is that if you don't distance yourself from them, not only may you find yourself miserable, but you are likely to repeat toxic patterns and cycles, especially if they are close to you.

I was terrible at determining what was making me unhappy, simply because I did not know what I wanted. The influence of my upbringing would bear down on me if ever I had to make my own decisions, which was seldom, because I would abdicate that responsibility whenever possible. I not only was paralyzed with indecision, but I also felt that I wasn't "allowed" to make the big decisions for myself. I couldn't decide what was important because I grew up to believe I wasn't worthy of having that responsibility, and so I allowed others to determine what should be important to me. The fact is, I hadn't grown up at all, and it wasn't until much later that I gave myself "permission" to take control of my life.

However, even in such a poor mental condition and a deprived emotional state, I still kept rebelling internally against any values or ideas being imposed on me. I kept hoping, fantasizing really, that I would get "my turn" to choose. In the absence of hope, fantasy was my only ally, but I had to start somewhere. From there, it built up, one thing upon another—fantasy, hope, identity, values—until I finally recognized for myself what mattered, and that I mattered. My learning was extremely slow, but important nonetheless. Learning is lifelong, so eventually finding your identity and creating your own values is an intrinsically important event in human development, however late it arrives. Keeping in mind what is important to you helps you to hone your instincts, so when something isn't working, you know when you need to work to repair it or to move on.

VALUES

Values are driven by identity. After all, how can you know what is important to you if you don't know who you are and what you want? Finding, testing and determining your own values are what defines you as an individual. It provides you the basis for making the decisions about how you want to live your life. This pursuit may require giving up old values that were once imposed upon you.

Life lessons lay the groundwork for finding out what is truly important to you. As you go through life, learning is continually happening with each experience, but it is not always at the same rate as everyone else or focused on the same things as some other people. Personal development was not in my orbit because it wasn't a recognized "thing" in my circle of influence when I was growing up, and I would never have recognized my need for it nor seen myself as deserving of it. I accepted whatever was right in front of me because my level of development simply didn't allow for me to "see" that far outside of myself. I was ignorant of the workings of the world around me and my place in it.

I provided no challenge, and I unquestioningly accepted the values that were given to me, employing coping strategies that helped keep me "safe" in what seemed an unsafe world, as I had unconsciously assimilated, until I was in my forties. If you have experienced this lack of personal interaction and growth, or even impairment, I will guide you to understand that no matter what level of development you are at, you can make significant, positive changes

to your life without making damaging alterations to your circumstances or derailing your life because of trauma (although in my
case, out of desperation, I decided that I needed to make sweeping
changes and a clean break). It can be done by altering your mindset,
experiencing your emotions, including pain, and adapting behaviors
to a new and improved set of criteria for including things in your life
and removing those which no longer serve you. Those criteria are
determined by your values.

EXAMINING YOUR VALUES

The values that you inherited from family, culture, religion and society can be accepted or challenged. Part of moving from childhood
to adulthood is deciding for yourself what you want and what is
important to you. At the beginning it is good to have an example of
values from others (usually family is the first influence) to help ori-
ent yourself in the world, in relation to others in society. Things like
sharing, obedience and friendship are "good" values that are often
instilled in children. As you grow and mature, it is desirable that
you learn to decide for yourself what is important. Often expectations from parents or others force you to adhere to values imposed
on you, in order to maintain familial and social bonds and to feel
a sense of belonging, which we human beings crave so much. At
maturity, in a supportive environment and in the absence of con-
trolling factors or restrictions (people or circumstances), you can
begin to determine your own values by the life lessons you have
learned through experience with others and by challenging old values when confronted with new information that aligns with your
experience. This is the process that you will take by examining your
own values and considering whether they work for you or not.

Values Exercise

Make a list of people (on paper, in a journal or use your smartphone if you prefer). Write next to each person who they are, or how they are related to you, and what kind of relationship you have with them—positive, negative or neutral. Leave a column free to include the values you inherited from them or their expectations of you. Then include another column for what your fears are. Try comparing the two lists and see if your fears line up with any of the values you were taught. Continue by journaling some answers to the following questions: Are your values inherited, or ones that you have developed yourself? What are they, and how are they working for you?

The lessons you have learned in life, probably through interactions with others, are what will inform your decisions to choose what to believe in or not. My problem was that my interactions were very limited with others, as I numbed and shut down. It not only prevented me from a larger, more full experience of life, but by shutting people out I had unknowingly prevented my own progression and also had shut down the process of development in general. My fear of not belonging, and not wanting to stand out or rock the boat, kept me from connecting with people, even my own family, and stemmed from nonexistent self-worth and a woeful lack of self-regard. My life was lacking in depth of experience and based out of fear, making it virtually impossible to develop any values of my own. I sought validation through others, because I valued their opinions over my own.

I was very lucky, though. I did have people who loved and cared for me (especially my husband and his family), but they were understandably clueless as to what I was going through and why. They could not fathom the reasons for my tendency to generally avoid interacting by seeking refuge in sleep, which was the only boundary I could manage to enforce during my depression. But I later learned from these experiences, however limited they were by my mental and emotional condition.

Even though it was slow and incremental, I did learn and progress by allowing myself to consider what was truly right for me and pushing the boundaries of accepted and expected behavior within my marriage. These things began to occur a little while before my divorce and meeting Myles, and from those lessons I figured out what was important to me, what my values were, plus what I would and would not allow to continue. As you look back on your life, it is important to discern which values are working for you and which ones aren't.

PAY ATTENTION TO THE RED FLAGS

A simple exercise of asking yourself questions will help you determine your values. "What do I want out of life?" and "How do I want to live?" are general but simple, all-encompassing questions that can help guide you toward your true self. The bigger question is this: "What is important to me?" The answer will give you the biggest indicator of whether your life is aligned with your values and whether you are experiencing authentic interactions guided by your true self. One thing to watch out for is to notice whether you continually find yourself attempting to live up to someone else's expectations. That is, living according to someone else's values. It can be hard to differentiate them from your own values, especially when you haven't defined for yourself what they are.

The next time something is asked or expected of you, remember to ask yourself, "Is this what I really want?" If not, pay attention to those red flags. I would imagine in my mind a red flag going up when I recognized something that didn't align with what I wanted. You may decide to help someone out, which is always your choice, and is helpful to maintain bonds, especially if you do so out of concern or care for another. Other times you have to do things that you don't want to do in life in order to pay the bills and so on, but that is not what I am talking about here. The things over which you do have control and you do have a choice are the things where you can practice differentiating from other people by stopping what you are begrudgingly doing solely for the sake of others and stating what is important to you.

It may seem difficult to do a sudden about-face with your family, but there are strategies to make it easier. Once you have created the awareness in yourself to notice the red flags, or to recognize the gut feeling that tells you to say no, then practice stopping the automatic reactions of "doing what you are told" or doing things mindlessly. First off, stop yourself from automatically saying yes to things. Just don't say anything at all except perhaps "wait," or "let me think." If it is hard for you to say no when asked to do something, prepare back-up statements to create new responses instead of letting "autopilot" take over. I used statements like "I wish I could help you out, but I can't right now," "Give me a minute to think about that" or "Let me get back to you on that," which gives you the mental space to figure out how you want to respond, especially if you are like me and need some time to think about what you want to say.

When you have mastered the use of these phrases and see the effect they have in getting you what you want, or addressing what you don't want, you can then extend it to something like "I don't know how I feel about that," or "That doesn't work for me," which are riskier in terms of response because you may be questioned why, so you will want to ease into those first, before moving onto other, more detailed responses that are relevant to your particular life situation. Having tools to get through these situations is the essential first step in asserting your needs, speaking your "truth" about what is important to you and creating those crucial personal values.

STRIP YOUR INFLUENCES

Taking away all familial, cultural, religious and romantic expectations or obligations, you will now examine what it is that you want in your life, by starting with a blank slate. What is important to you outside of the things mentioned above? It's quite an exercise to mentally strip yourself of your influences, but it is part of the process of rebuilding yourself from the ground up. You must take away everything derived from others and figure out what remains. What is left is your essence.

Ask yourself the following questions:

- Without family, who are you?
- Without your partner, who is left?
- Without religious affiliation, who is at your core? Who is at the seat of your soul?
- What do you do, or what do you feel like, when you are alone?
- Do you fantasize about what you really want to do with your time?
- Are there things that interest you that you have long forgotten or given up?
- Has your upbringing forbidden you from doing things that you love?
- Have you yourself deemed something you like not worthwhile because it won't make you money or please a parent or partner?
- Is there something you always wanted to do but won't allow yourself to do it?
- Do you secretly hate something that you grew up doing and continue to do?
- Is there a way of being that you would prefer over how you are living now?

Once you have recognized the aspects of your core being, of your true self, the values you acquired from childhood can be kept or discarded according to whether they align with your desires.

You can choose whether any of those values are still important to you by examining them objectively, without any external influence, which gives you a bit of distance from your circumstances in order to decide upon the merit of those values.

In some cases, values handed down are rather subtle or opaque, so it may take some time to identify them. For instance, getting your chores done or respecting your elders may be values you absorbed, whether or not those chores were fair and age-appropriate or the elders in your life deserved that unilateral respect. Basically, take each item or topic and ask yourself if it is something you want in your life. By temporarily removing from yourself all inherited values, you can add back into your consciousness that which is important to you, therefore creating your values from scratch.

Doing this work of identifying your values means you actually embody the things that have meaning for you. Ask yourself what is important to you? What is a must-do or must-have element in your life? In terms of must-haves, try to think of it as maintaining what you have rather than what you are going to get. For example, if your goal is that the personal relationship you already have is transformed from one filled with strife into one that is mutually satisfying, and in which you feel cherished, this is something that may be more worthwhile to investigate, say by attending counseling, rather than throwing away your relationship. Sometimes though, you must make changes, even drastic ones, in order to get what you want.

THE ROLE OF HOPE

Hope is a useful tool for keeping forward momentum in your journey. Instilling hope is a process that results from your hard work that was done in the previous chapters. Being able to assimilate all the information from the exercises and learning from them can boost your confidence. That boost in confidence can translate to making life goals and seeking more opportunities, whether for jobs, relationships or new activities. This makes more room for purpose and passion to enter your life. You create the mental space to have faith in a better future, while creating new opportunities and to participate in life.

I'm not talking about wishful thinking either. Things are not going to magically fall from the sky. You will need to go out and participate in the world to discover new opportunities. Fixating on a thing that you don't have can also lead you astray from the journey of self-discovery that you are on, so keep goals relevant to what is in your life now, and then you can pursue grander or more risky goals (in terms of attainability) later, after you have built up some confidence by seeing and evaluating the results from your efforts.

WHAT ARE YOUR GOALS?

As a visioning exercise, ask yourself, what are your goals? Where do you see yourself a year from now, and what do you hope to achieve? This can be as complex or as simple as you please, but do spend some time journaling about these questions, and formalize your goals from this journaling. As you rework your values, you will transform yourself from a person fractured by competing desires from others into someone who is an integrated whole. When I first left my marriage, my main concern was making a better living to support my two children, so I applied and was accepted at my local university, after a grueling schedule of volunteer work, I might add, which was a prerequisite for application. Before entering school that September, I began going out to clubs with my friend to finally pursue my passion for dancing, which I never allowed myself to do while in my marriage. Unfortunately, the COVID-19 pandemic shut that down, but it allowed me some time to consider what other things I wanted to pursue.

I tried, and failed miserably, at financial investing, but at least it was my failure, and I own it. Funny enough, I actually trust myself more now because of that failure than if I had never tried, if I had feared the worst and let it stop me from trying. I did, however, write a book (*flaunts shamelessly*), so I now know that I can live according to my own desires and values, as well as live up to my potential. Identifying and living according to your own values is imperative to creating personal autonomy. You must have personal autonomy in order to change your behavior. That autonomy is exercised when you are able to achieve goals on your own, through your own effort, which is owing to the work you did determining your values and the areas in which you prefer to spend your time.

Hope begins to blossom where little or none was before, once you realize that it is completely within your power to live according to your own desires and dictates, and that change is possible. Previous efforts to evaluate and decide what is important to you will point the way toward purpose as you move forward in this journey. As you will learn, finding your purpose is actually less work and more fun.

7
Change: How Can I Do That?

THIS IS THE chapter where you bring all that you've learned together and then put it all into practice. Doing the exercises from previous chapters are the experiences that will stimulate the all-important, integrating effect of wholeness, which will steer you toward happiness and ultimately lead you to personal power. This is not a linear path, however. Your progression depends on how you use what you've been taught, shown and provided in terms of lessons and exercises. Spend your time on what works best for you first, or is the easiest to achieve, and which aspects of the work you find the most valuable or effective. Start with those areas, but consider going back to do the other exercises too because they can work better together.

I initially did physical practices such as yoga and some belly-dance long before I was on the healing path in my forties. I also tried parkour (If you don't know what this is, check out David Belle and Sebastien Foucan online—*amazing!*) and I have been a cyclist for many years. As an adult, I played soccer, did weight training and went hiking on occasion, among other things, so I had a number of physical outlets that, unbeknownst to me, began the healing process.

One of the things I almost never allowed myself to do until much later, however, is dance. It was frowned upon by my husband, so I did not take up belly dancing until my thirties and virtually never went out to clubs to dance. I tried out or returned to some of these embodiment practices later, specifically for the purpose of healing myself after recognizing their significance. The physicality of these activities and endeavors was the way in which much of the years of repressed emotion and built-up tension in my body was released. It took a *long* time, though.

Supplied with the knowledge of what you are doing and why, and purposefully using it to help you let go of past wounds, you will take off years of fumbling in the dark to resolve your trauma. Pick something that you like and that you can do without feeling any pressure to perform. Make it fun to keep the momentum going, but most of all, be present in that time you set aside for yourself. Consider it part of your healing, because it most certainly is. The key is practice. Keep doing it, and do it because it feels good.

Then broaden your practices to include ones that may be important to you but that may fall outside what I have described here, such as medical care, religious or spiritual practice, meditation, psychology and counseling, and so on. Treating yourself holistically with a full range of approaches will help integrate and connect your healing with what is important in your life or particularly helpful in your journey. Integration of self is the goal so that you can be present for others. When you are connected to yourself and your own needs, your ability to connect and truly attune to others' needs will guide you to a more integrated life, full of possibility.

MIND-BODY CONNECTION

Trying new things may seem trivial in terms of healing, and if you are in the emotional muck of the healing process, it may not be the time to take on a new challenge. Eventually you will need to integrate physical practices with treatments for the psyche because trauma affects all of these areas. Releasing emotion through crying or yelling (in a safe and private environment) may be necessary first, in order to discharge emotional energy. Rest is also an important part of healing, even if it is an internal process. Not only do muscles need to rest and recover, but so does your mind, your heart and your soul.

I had to lie on the couch in front of the fire for months to recover from the wreckage of my childhood emotional neglect, the denial of the impact of it on my life and the trauma of my heartbreak, which replicated my childhood rejection and abandonment issues. All of these things had combined, characterized and encapsulated my trauma. You may not have the energy to put toward physical tasks and undertakings right now, and that is okay. When you are ready for it, absolutely do it, but until then, rest and recover, or cry and scream. Ultimately it is up to you to determine what works for you, your family context, your environment, your comfort level and what stage you are at in the process.

SOMATIC HEALING

Somatic (body-based) healing involves the mind-body connection. I have focused a lot on the concept of embodiment because of its effectiveness. I use the idea of somatic healing as a guide because physical activity was such an important part of my journey. While I am familiar with and can offer some of the concepts of somatic healing here, there is a specific therapy called somatic experiencing, created by Dr. Peter Levine, that goes deeper than the information that I have provided here and for which counseling is a part of the process. Somatic healing and somatic experiencing are therapies that are carried out by trained professionals with whom you work in partnership, and who guide you specifically, which I cannot do in a book. Seek a local professional for this type of therapy if it interests you.

There are also other therapeutic options that make connections between mind and body. There is a reason that expressive arts such as painting, acting, dancing and music (playing or singing) are involved in healing. They work in concert with physical recreation, involvement in things like yoga, meditation, massage and breath work, and can even be considered physical themselves because they, of course, use the body as their conduit. Physical and creative practices can unlock trapped energies in the body from years of repression, suppression, denial, anxiety and fear. Where do you think those energies go when, as a child, you experience these emotions and reactions, especially if you had no outlet to express them, out of fear of your parents' reactions? The energy stays with you, coiled up inside you like a snake ready to strike, in every muscle, every fiber, every tissue, waiting for the chance to unleash years of pent-up emotion like anger or fear on the world. This can be extremely cathartic, but uncontrolled and messy, as in my case, to say nothing of the potential to harm others if left unaddressed.

BREATH AND VOCAL WORK

Practicing breathwork helps dispel unconscious fear through the physical act of breathing, which promotes more oxygen flow to the brain and allows clearer thinking. It also helps with calming those fears by training your response to be one of conscious calm instead of instant alarm. Executive functions such as emotional regulation occur in the neocortex, which evolved as the newest structure of the brain, while the fight, flight, freeze or fawn response originates in the amygdala, the oldest, most primitive part of the brain. Breathwork is an effective counter to the instinctive response of the nervous system of fight, flight, freeze or fawn. You can practice another breathing exercise by training your attention on the breath by counting for four seconds while breathing in through your nose, holding for five seconds and then breathing out for seven seconds through the mouth. Clearing your thoughts while doing this is a good starting point. Later, you can try focusing on an uncomfortable situation such as confronting someone with what you want to say, which may upset them. This will help you to hone the skill of communication while also making yourself heard, which leads us to vocal work.

Vocal work provides life-affirming self-validation with the practice of using your voice. This is especially powerful if you have remained silent for much of your history, struggling with the ability to even speak. It is a way to rehearse what you want to say, to get used to using your voice, literally and figuratively, for it is a practice in which you actually demand that your voice be heard in the world, after a lifetime of feeling unworthy. Practice the below exercise with your partner, a trusted family member or close friend to say what you want to say to someone else but have been having difficulty in doing so. Tell your helper what you really feel, as if they were the person at issue. Starting with "I" statements, such as "I feel this way when you ..." helps it to be less confrontational.

If you're having trouble with this, start by adopting phrases like, "I've been wanting to say this for a long time, but I need time to gather my thoughts" or "Give me a minute to think" or perhaps, "Can we book a time to discuss this issue? I need to prepare what I want to say," before getting right into it, in order to give yourself the time you need to mentally and emotionally prepare, even if you're only with your helper for now. It is yet another way to practice expansion, by allowing self-expression and acknowledging your own acceptance of yourself as a worthy participant in life.

If you get hampered by not wanting to upset anyone and then end up taking on the feelings yourself, you may have internalized this response from childhood, with the outcome of your trauma having likely molded your psyche in this way. A combination of physical, spiritual, social and emotional practices can help free this emotional blockage or alter your reactivity, by creating and encouraging expansion. Physical expansion of the muscles, the diaphragm, ligaments, tendons and even organs, can in turn promote emotional expansion, which creates room to feel emotions, especially those that are long forgotten and buried in the subconscious, which your inner child has purposefully hidden away in order to protect you. This happened when your inner child had no understanding of— and no practical way of dealing with—an event or the actions of the caregiver or authority figure at hand.

This is what gets trapped in the body and mind, and ultimately, the soul of the individual. It forms the emerging character of the person by altering the traits of the individual, at a basic, fundamental level, and requires a great deal of focus and determination to change in later years. It is when the adult gets curious about how they came to become who they are (as a best-case scenario, or they finally fall apart emotionally in ignorance of their plight) that they can undertake the challenge of getting to know themselves and begin to get acquainted with the real individual inside, instead of just the idealized fantasy of who they want to be, or may have always intended to be, but didn't know how to achieve it. Physical practices help to facilitate the kind of opening and expansion that is required for the expression of self, even verbally.

Another reason I keep circling back to physical practices is that it not only releases pent-up energy and emotion, but it also helps point you toward your interests. This is what can steer you toward your purpose. I'm not saying taking up kickboxing means you are destined to be the next MMA champion, but maybe if you already have a background in it, you can teach classes at your local community center, volunteer with children and youth or participate in local competitions to get some satisfaction out of your practice. Or you can just do it for your own personal satisfaction or sense of achievement. Perhaps you have already tried other pursuits and have enjoyed their benefits. If your awareness has already led you to doing the things that give you some life satisfaction, great! It can create a feeling of personal fulfillment, or maybe kickstart a drive toward community connection or even altruism, which can have corollary benefits for your psyche while simultaneously releasing trapped emotional energy in your body. The point is that you will be getting something out of life, and maybe even be able to give something back.

If you have been holding yourself back for a number of years, taking on a new challenge can give you a sense of accomplishment. It has the potential to turn into a life's purpose, simply by doing it, because you could discover a passion for volunteer work (of any kind), or it may open doors to other pursuits you never considered by introducing you to new people and new ideas that never occurred to you before. You can change the direction of your life by getting off the couch, while simultaneously experiencing catharsis from the removal of emotional blockage that such focused movement promotes.

It also assists in differentiation, a hallmark of maturity, which was something I lacked. I just transferred my tendency to acquiesce to authority from my parents onto my husband, even though I did physically move out of my parents' home. Differentiating (separating oneself mentally, emotionally and often physically from your caregivers) usually begins in adolescence, but it came extremely late for me. It was when I left my marriage that I took the first step toward becoming myself and living life on my own terms.

HOLISTIC CARE

It is important to consider the whole person when treating trauma. Holistic wellness approaches to therapy are becoming increasingly accepted as forms of treatment, by considering the whole person rather than just a set of symptoms. Traditional Western medicine can often overlook the totality of the person by treating the symptoms of illness with prescriptions, and perhaps some exercise or physical therapies such as chiropractic, massage and physiotherapy, to name a few. The body can succumb to illness because of hidden stressors and causes, and the person is often only medicated for physical relief and the soul is neglected altogether.

The conclusion is that any mental and emotional problems fall under the umbrella of psychology, and so are left to psychologists and counselors to discover and treat. Alternative medicine also offers treatments specific to one discipline or area, such as Traditional Chinese Medicine (TCM), naturopathic medicine, acupuncture or seeing a dietician, and while each is important, they are still not treating you as a whole person. A holistic approach to trauma would include either all or many of the above practitioners working simultaneously, perhaps even with clergy, which would consider the spirit along with the body and mind. That is, the physical symptoms as well as the mental, emotional, spiritual and overall wellness of the individual would be considered.

As an exercise, reflect on all of the areas of your life that you think would be helpful to your healing, and match them to an activity that interests you. The broad scope of these aspects of yourself can be explored through a physical activity, a body-based practice, a spiritual practice or even a creative one. This way, any one of them can take the lead in your healing.

For me, it was my body that took the lead and not by my choice. It was losing control at that funeral that finally awakened me to the fact that my life was way out of whack and that my mind, body and spirit were not aligned. Five years ago, my body intelligence took over and said to me, *You are not getting the message, so this will get your attention.* Boom! Emotional breakdown. It took five years to discover my trauma, experience my traumatic response and subsequently to heal from it.

The tragedy of my emotional neglect was I did not recognize it, and I carried it throughout my life like a burden on my back, with no understanding of its origins nor any inkling that I needed help or had anything to heal. It held me back in all areas of my life and kept me from recognizing my needs, all the while conspiring to keep me from connecting to anyone, least of all myself. Trauma left me alone, clueless as to how to look after myself emotionally, and inhibiting my ability to successfully interact or connect with others, which is the touchstone of society and the essence of humanity.

CONNECTION

The most important connection, of course, is the connection to self. Without this, you will be hard-pressed to benefit from the full spectrum of emotional connection that is possible with others. Nurturing a connection to yourself is critical, and this is what I have encouraged throughout this book by doing the exercises to create a sense of calm, clear understanding of your identity and, ultimately, your purpose. The concepts lead you to an integration of yourself through the process of discovering the missing links to your wholeness and happiness and allowing you to work on repairing or replacing those links. I came up with a radical idea to bring together all aspects of my healing work and practice. Naturally, my final act of integration took the form of dance. I decided that I would invite my inner child to dance, to show her that I indeed loved her first and foremost, and to make that most intimate of connections: to myself.

I played one of my favorite pieces of music, which had the rhythm of a waltz, one-two-three, one-two-three. I held up my hands to lead, and once I internally felt her "accept" the invitation by taking my hand, I led her in a most passionate dance. We twirled and spun with reckless abandon. As the song neared its end, I felt an unexpected change that happened quite organically and was both undeniable and magical in its implications. As I brought in my extended arms, enfolding them around me in an embrace while I danced, I felt the two of us dissolve into each other and truly become one. In that moment, I was finally able to connect to my true self. I was able to integrate my inner child and my entire life's experiences into the person I was now, and I wept at length.

I later realized that it reminded me of the one time when I danced with my father at a cousin's wedding. As I stood on his feet while we waltzed, I felt shy and awkward as this was the only time outside of being very young that I remember sharing an intimate experience with him. I made the emotional connection that it was this moment that I was revisiting, reenacting and now replacing with my own intimate dance. Talk about integration.

My stories and examples are extreme, I realize. You don't need to take the exact same path as I did to make this work for you. In fact, it probably won't make sense to you to do the same things as me, because for starters, dance may not be your thing. However, my experience illustrates that you need to step outside of your comfort zone to get results. Like I said, this journey requires courage. Otherwise, you're just holding back and wasting your own time. Not committing to do the work to change your circumstances is equivalent to going through the motions. It's a slippery slope to slide back into old habits, or to procrastinate and put it off. It is akin to spinning your wheels but staying in one spot. Lack of progress will be inevitable, and you will continue to hurt yourself.

Presenting yourself in a way that fits into others' ideas of who you should be (or pretending to be someone else for their benefit) disintegrates your sense of self, which is counterproductive and toxic to your well-being. The result of being confident in who you actually are is that you connect with others because you are presenting your true self to the world, which people respond to naturally and spontaneously. Being yourself has the benefit of people around you reacting to who you really are and responding authentically, so that you know you are genuinely connecting on a basic level, the most elementary level of your being, when getting to know someone. It allows you to develop a sense of the natural rhythm of interaction among people, which may have been absent in your process of growth. Generally, it helps make you comfortable with others because you have developed comfort with yourself, and this quality is evident to others, making you a more positive, self-assured person and therefore more approachable.

Ultimately, this work allows you to develop your intuition, once you have tuned in to your own wants and needs and shifted away from trying to meet the perceived wants and needs of others in order to gain acceptance, nurturance and love from them. Once you are able to direct your own life toward a path of your own choosing, and using your own desires as guidance for yourself, your intuition can help you with decision-making. It not only allows you to pursue what you feel passionate about, but it also makes it so that you can strengthen your current and future relationships, because your care for others is real concern for their well-being, instead of stemming from a need to care for them in the hope of being loved and accepted by them in return.

I'm not suggesting that you don't already truly care for your loved ones, or that reciprocation of love and care are not important parts of a relationship. It's just that the driving force behind your actions comes from an internal motivator, instead of being incentivized by others externally. Once you have a handle on this idea and you recognize that your motivations derive from your care and concern for others, your actions are changed to being motivated by your ability and willingness to help and care for others. This is opposed to doing it as a way to seek love, affection or favor, out of fear and anxiety. When you are responding out of love instead of fear, you are displaying your true self and your true nature.

Your intuition naturally develops as a result of how your true nature tells you to respond. You learn to trust not only yourself but also your ability to determine what is best for you, and your learning continues to expand. You then learn to trust others, which is diametrically opposed to the fear-based patterns you developed as a child that previously served as a means of protection. Moving away from these old patterns is another form of expansion.

When your inner (private/personal/internal) and outer realities (external life circumstances) match, you have achieved a sort of oneness, or unity of the soul with self. This can allow a connection to a community of people that you otherwise were unable to access before, because people cannot respond to you when you turn inward or socially withdraw. Having this new set of skills allows for better connection with others, because you are relaxed about who you are as a person and no longer fret about who you present to the world in an effort to please others. When you present yourself unabashedly, unapologetically to the world, people respond differently to you. Some respond very positively, others may still reject you, but the rejection doesn't have the same sting as before. It is easier to accept that not everyone will be your friend, and you pay close attention to those who are your true allies, friends and of course "family," whether you are related or not.

Connectedness is the ultimate goal of humanity, regardless of its source and whether or not there is a spiritual component for you. Connectedness is so important, as belonging is an inborn biological instinct. Learning to connect with others is worth the effort of making changes to your life, if connection is lacking in your life, as it was for me. Connectedness not only has social benefits, but it also taps into our deepest needs. Connectedness forms the basis of the human experience. I believe it is not only felt on a personal level, but it is also experienced on a universal level, in terms of energetic vibration.

SPIRITUALITY AND TRAUMA

I think that spirituality and the experience of healing from trauma are closely linked. I know that may sound very "out there" or "woo-woo" to those who don't have spiritual beliefs, or at least not those matching more metaphysical types of spirituality. However, my point is not actually based in scripture or religious dogma of any kind but in both theoretical and recognized science. Every living thing on earth gives off a magnetic field. Plants and animals (including humans) are all able to sense and respond to those "waves" or "vibrations," which is the energy that I've referred to previously.

The Scientific and Medical Network (2016) states that "It is apparent that there is enough evidence to suggest that human energy fields exist and that they carry information for growth and repair. These fields appear to be at two levels—an electromagnetic field that interfaces with the physical body (Burr and Becker) and an etheric field or magneto-electric field (Reid and Steiner)." The World Health Organization (2016) supports this: "Low-frequency magnetic fields induce circulating currents within the human body. The strength of these currents depends on the intensity of the outside magnetic field. If sufficiently large, these currents could cause stimulation of nerves and muscles or affect other biological processes." The U.S. National Library of Medicine, National Institutes of Health (2020) also confirms that "We evolutionarily inherited vibrational sensitivity, which is hard-wired in our body and brain," while T. Hunt in *Scientific American* (2021) adds that "Vibrations, resonance, are the key mechanism behind human consciousness, as well as animal consciousness more generally."

Granted, these brief descriptions of physical phenomena don't unequivocally prove that this is the explanation for connection, consciousness and spirituality. But they definitely recognize that there are senses beyond our five main ones that we all share, and there is a potential case for connection on a physical, quantum level. The work of Dr. Bruce Lipton, PhD, particularly resonates with me (the puns never cease) because it ties in spirituality with physics, biology—particularly in the field of epigenetics—and quantum mechanics. Those so-called "vibes" that people give off are real alterations to the magnetic field, based on the energy they emit. You can unconsciously and subconsciously influence the "vibes" you send out.

According to Dr. Lipton in the 2020 production *Inner Evolution* on Gaia, "Constructive interference … is also recognized in our life experience as good vibes and so, when you're in that field, the energy around you is interfering with you in a constructive manner and as a result, you are feeling more energy. Good vibes. Vibes are the source of life. Energy is the source of life." He continues to say, "The primary language on this planet is vibration reading. Vibration can enhance your life and save you from any problems that destructive interference would have caused. It's important to recognize the vital nature of reading energy fields, so vital that every organism on this planet creates its life based on reading these fields. And everything generates fields." Constructive interference, of course, refers to the good vibes that are felt during positive, life-affirming interactions with people. Destructive interference means the bad vibes you experience when you are dealing with someone's negative, toxic energy or someone whose energy simply doesn't "align" or "vibe" with you. By tuning in to your and others' energy, you are tuned in to life.

Once you are more attuned to your true self, you present yourself in a way that people are more likely to respond positively to. Attunement to yourself also allows better attunement to others, so caring for your loved ones becomes a much easier task, because you are responding to their actual needs rather than what you perceive their needs to be. You are better able to hear what people are actually saying rather than listening to them through the filter of your own fears and doubts. In short, attunement to others fosters connection, which positively influences your "vibes." Being able to respond to others by not only "being yourself" but also allowing others to be themselves makes you a better human being. In short, learning about yourself will make you better able to help others, or to serve, which is one of the highest callings of humanity.

Chapter 7 References

Web Team/The Scientific and Medical Network (2016). The human energy field. Published online April 2, 2016. Retrieved (2021) from https://explore.scimednet.org/index.php/2016/04/02/the-human-energy-field/

World Health Organization (2016). *Radiation: Electromagnetic fields.* Newsroom. Q & A Detail. Published online August 4, 2016. Retrieved (2021) from https://www.who.int/news-room/q-a-detail/radiation-electromagnetic-fields

PMC/US National Library of Medicine/National Institutes of Health (2020). Vibration detection: Its function and recent advances in medical applications. Published online June 17, 2020. doi: 10.12688/f1000research.22649.1 Retrieved (2021) from https://www.ncbi.nlm.nih.gov/pmc/articles/PMC7308885/

Hunt, T. (2018). The hippies were right: It's all about vibrations, man! A new theory of consciousness. *Scientific American.* Published online December 5, 2018. Retrieved (2021) from https://blogs.scientificamerican.com/observations/the-hippies-were-right-its-all-about-vibrations-man/

Gaia Inc. (2020). Inner Evolution. *It's a matter of energy.* Season 1, Episode 4. Aired March 30, 2020. Retrieved (2021).

8

Reflect: What Have I Learned from All of This?

IN THIS CHAPTER, I will guide you to use reflection to integrate all that you have learned so far. You will take what you have learned about yourself through becoming aware and begin to transform yourself from the inside out. It requires a willingness to look back with honesty on what your life was, and is now, without judgment, while acknowledging what you will need to work on in order to create the future that you want. You can reflect on things that will be most effective for guiding you in your personal journey. Staying present is one of the most beneficial practices you can learn. It keeps you grounded by reminding you that now is what is truly important. Learning to trust after the failure of your caregivers to meet your needs is difficult but vital. Trust, especially in yourself, can finally form after integrating all the lessons you have learned into your experience, once the massive build-up of your fears is dispelled and the unresolved trauma is released from your psyche. Learning to let go of blame, to let go of expectations and to let go of emotional baggage that doesn't serve you anymore provides such cathartic freedom that personal power is the natural result.

PRESENCE

The present moment is all that we have. No matter how much work you do to resolve your trauma and exorcise the ghosts of your past, you really only have how you are thinking, feeling and acting right now to show for your efforts. There is no need to judge yourself for how far you have come on your journey, or to endlessly ruminate on what you could have done differently. This is pointless and a waste of your precious energy. You are here, now, doing what you can to better your circumstances and showing up as your best self in order to manifest positive change in your life. Finding contentment in simply being, with no timetables, external goals or expectations to be met is what paves the way for peace. Using a mindfulness practice can move you toward that sense of peace.

Mindfulness is the best practice for keeping yourself in the present moment. Continually reminding yourself that what is happening right now is of the utmost importance keeps you grounded and in the present moment, banishing the thought of all that has passed before now and releasing the wishes, expectations or worries of what might be in the future. The past is the past, and the future may be completely and utterly different from what you expect, so learning to recognize, accept and enjoy the present moment is the best way to appreciate your life and live it to the fullest. It also often takes the form of practice. For instance, during those times when you go down the rabbit hole of doubt, or fall back into the habit of negative self-talk, you can remind yourself in the here and now to challenge the reality or the truth of those statements. Another practice you can try is meditation.

Meditation can be used as a mindfulness practice, and it is well-known for its ability to create ease and peace in your being by negotiating perceived mental or emotional obstacles in a gentle way. Instead of trying to forcefully "empty your mind," as is often thought of meditation, you let thoughts appear naturally, but then take a stance of observing them objectively, almost as if they aren't yours or they are just objects floating in your mind, and use your imagination to gently move them aside or, if it is helpful, put them inside of a box. There is no judgment about these thoughts, and they become devoid of emotional content by taking this objective approach, allowing yourself to detach from your thoughts. The time spent in meditation benefits your health by changing brain waves from a more active pattern to one of more relaxation, which is why it is so powerful in helping to achieve calm stillness. As always, if this activity is too intense for you, stop, and use the breathing and grounding exercises provided in Chapter 1 to come back to equilibrium.

Guided Visualization Exercise

If you have not meditated before, you can practice with the simple guided visualization meditation I provide here or, if you prefer, you can try going online to find free guided visualization meditations or simple relaxation videos with sound or music and imagery.

In this "healing screen" guided visualization, you will filter out old energy and tension.

Begin by making yourself comfortable. Gently close your eyes if that is comfortable for you or, if you prefer, simply lower your gaze. Take a few moments to settle yourself.

If at any time in this meditation you feel uncomfortable or strong emotions arise, please practice self-care and pause the meditation or try a different meditation.

Take a deep breath. And allow your body to relax. Breathe slowly and deeply.

Feel your abdomen rise and fall with each breath. Take your time. Be gentle. Allow yourself to let go of the external world.

As you breathe, expand your breath into your entire tor-so. Feel your abdomen rise and fall and your lungs ex-pand with each breath. Be conscious of how you breathe; breathe slowly, gently.

Relax your face muscles and your scalp.

Relax your shoulders and neck.

Relax your arms and your hands.

Be ever so patient and gentle with yourself. Relax your feet and legs.

Breathe and let all be at peace within you.

Let's begin the journey to the Healing Screen.

I invite you to imagine that you are in a bright, beautiful hallway. Using your mind's eye, you descend down a grand, spiral stairway. Feel each step you take. At the bottom of the stairway there is magnificent, grand doorway. The double doors are gilded and slowly open before you, welcoming you as you approach. You step through the doorway into a beautiful garden. You walk along the path of this garden, admiring the trees, flowers and birds. You notice your favorite flowers and pause to smell their lovely aroma. You take a moment to enjoy the comforting sounds of a trickling stream.

See yourself at the entrance to a lovely trail leading into the forest. It looks inviting and welcomes you. The trees around you are very old and tall, and the sun shines through their leaves, providing just enough warmth to make you feel comfortable. As you walk along the path, twigs crunch under your feet. You hear birds chirping in the distance and hear the rustle of the leaves in the soft breeze. You begin to feel a oneness with nature.

You arrive at a clearing in the forest. The clearing is lit from above with the soft, gentle light of the sun. It is very peaceful here. As you look around, you are drawn to a structure about 30 feet in front of you. You decide to walk over to it to get a better look. Along the way, you walk past a calm pond. It has leaves floating upon the water's surface.

When you reach the structure, you gaze upon it with wonder. It is a tall screen, in the shape and size of a large doorway. The screen is a healing, glistening, intricate silver mesh. As you stand in front of it, you feel it welcome you. This healing screen filters out what no longer serves you—anxiety, tension, worry or discomfort. It asks you to walk through it. Slowly, you take a step into the screen, then commit yourself by walking through it with confidence and intention. As you walk through it, you feel a slight resistance; this resistance is natural. It is the old energy that no longer serves you being filtered out of your body. You look back at the screen and notice a grayish deposit left on the screen. You already feel lighter and more clear-headed.

You walk around to the front of the screen, and walk through it again. Really feel the resistance as you walk through it.

Now, continue to walk through the screen, several more times. Each time, you become clearer and begin to glow with light, as more and more of the old energy is filtered out from your body. Take your time as you purify yourself over the next few minutes of quiet time.

Now you feel very light, clear and free from all anxiety, tension and worry or discomfort that you had before.

You approach the front of the screen, and with your hands you scoop up the grayish deposits toward the center of the screen, and lift it off the screen. This deposit feels heavy and sticky.

You now need to dispose of this deposit into the pond. You carry it over to the pond and toss it in, hearing the splash as it hits the surface, and you watch it sink down to the bottom of the pond and fully disappear. You immerse your hands in the cool water to cleanse them, and it feels so good.

It is now time to say thank you to the healing screen and walk back along the path through the forest to the garden, coming back to the gilded double doors. The doors open for you, welcoming you back. You see the grand spiral stairway, and start to ascend the stairs. As you reach the top of the stairs, you feel clear, calm and wonderful.

You realize that you are exactly how you are supposed to be right in this moment and that you are enjoying this present moment, this wonderful moment.

You may now gently move your hands and your feet, and open your eyes when you are ready.

If you want to go deeper into learning about mindfulness meditation or become a mindfulness facilitator, check out the work of Wendy Quan at www.TheCalmMonkey.com, a leading Mindfulness Meditation Facilitator Training & Certification program.

PLAN FOR SUCCESS

Congratulate yourself for taking this time to devote to yourself. It is not easy to carve out time in your busy life for this practice, let alone to do the other work in this book. Know that by taking the time to work on yourself by planning ahead, which is a strategy originating in the present, you allow yourself to leave the work for another specified time while you attend to other priorities that require your attention. Committing to any or all of the practices and exercises in this book will help you to build trust in your own ability to surmount the challenges you face in healing yourself, as well as in the healing process itself.

TRUST

Trust is critical for coming into your own power; ultimately, it starts with you. Trusting yourself is the most crucial act to living a life in which you are free to explore, free to move with confidence and free to love. Trust is the basis for love, which is fostered by empathy and nurtured with intimacy. Trust allows you to let down your guard, to be true to yourself by being especially mindful of your needs and boundaries, and to share yourself with others without fear, which is why it is so difficult to attain for those who have suffered emotional neglect.

Trust requires you to be vulnerable with someone else (despite your fears), in order to create relationships. This is why it is not only important and beneficial but actually easier to build a relationship with yourself first. You're not taking as big a risk by yourself, so the advantage is that you don't have to be as vulnerable as you would be with another person. However, being honest with yourself about your personal life circumstances may prove to be very challenging. You may deeply mistrust yourself, which is understandable, since getting needs met was a seemingly impossible task, as you craved and searched for validation outside of yourself while never believing yourself to have any worth. This is the perfect combination for an entrenched lack of trust in oneself and others, such as mine was. You must trust yourself fully to be able to heal from your trauma. In order to build trust in yourself, there are some specific things you can do.

Solo Trust Exercise

To start, try this exercise. Choose a place to stand somewhere in your home, and then close your eyes. Keeping eyes closed, find your way through your dwelling, going from room to room, feeling walls and door frames if necessary. Move around your home, identifying each room as you enter. (Please use caution, as this may be treacherous if you have stairs, lots of furniture to navigate, or items on the ground like kids' toys.) Go at whatever speed is comfortable, and take whatever precautions are necessary to feel safe enough to do this activity. You might occasionally bump into something, but try to have a sense of humor about it. The whole point is to learn to trust yourself, so staying safe from injury is actually part of the process, but accepting the "bumps" along the way is also tied to the process and a reminder of reality. See if you can go through one level of your home; stairs are not recommended.

This exercise is an illustration of learning to trust in the process. In terms of the work outlined in this book, using your memories as guides, you must trust that the memory is vivid for a reason, and trust your gut that it is important to examine the meaning of those recollections. Doing the physical practices gets you in tune with your body so that you can trust that the body's intelligence (its ability to continue performing, to discharge or release tension effectively through exercise or activity, and to tell you when something is wrong, through aches, pains, anxiety, panic or, yes, even a breakdown) will guide you toward the necessary steps in the healing process, all in the service of creating your best self.

I had to learn to trust not only myself but also to trust in the journey and to trust that life was going to be okay. You must build up to being able to trust others. For years and years, I didn't trust anyone or anything. I just stumbled along, dealing with whatever life threw at me. Now I fully embrace all the experiences that may arise in the course of my life, without fear or worry, and with trust that life will work itself out and that there are many connections to be made with people and many things left to be experienced. Once you have trust, you can accept the inherent risks that love and change entail. You can open yourself up to so much more, and your world expands accordingly in response to this opening of your soul to the possibilities that this world has to offer and the potential with the people that surround you. This is the power of trust and living a life guided by love instead of fear.

LETTING GO

Letting go is the result of trusting that the journey will result in the creation of your best self, and that is attained through staying present. Learning to let go is powerful. For me, it provided a sense of relief, and of peace, even though I still felt I had work to do. Letting go is the final step in the healing process, which will continue until you die. This will allow you to live your best life, because you won't be ruled by things that are out of your control. You can manage your anxieties through mindful practices, which help to remind you of all your blessings and aid in letting go of expectations and being happy despite less-than-ideal circumstances that are bound to arise in life. That is why I emphasize the idea of practice.

You ultimately choose how much, or in what way(s), you want to practice, but it is this disciplined approach to your own healing that will have the most impact. For your mind, body and soul to experience the necessary shifts that represent your learning, your mindset changes and your overall evolution, mindful practice is required. It can keep you present, help you trust the process and aid in learning to let go of expectations of yourself and of others. This is how personal power is gained. When you no longer have triggers that keep you entrenched in emotional warfare with yourself, and you are grateful and mindful of both your blessings and your challenges, you are powerful. It makes you unafraid of, well, almost anything. You now can take on whatever challenge or opportunity comes your way. This is where purpose comes in. More than that, it creates room for passion to blossom.

Your purpose and your passion may or may not be the same thing, but in this journey, whatever you end up discovering about yourself and what you want, both your purpose and your passion are going to be aligned with who you truly are and your deepest desires. Your purpose will have a direct antecedent in the connections you have made with people, whether it is reestablishing or rekindling past connections or gaining new ones. You may find purpose in how you serve others, relate with others or present ideas to others. Passion may also be connected to your relationships, but things like creativity and engagement, even in solo pursuits, are still important because the most important relationship is, of course, the one you have with yourself. You must sustain this relationship first and foremost before you can create—and sustain—relationships with other people. This is why even creative passions that are done alone have their place, because you must nurture your own soul before you can nurture others and maintain those relationships in your life.

Many realizations come with this healing work and with experience. My experience was such that I had to go through a trauma reenactment of rejection and abandonment with the love of my life, mimicking that which I felt with my father, in order to fully understand the healing process. The last day I saw Myles was when he communicated that he didn't love me anymore, and it tapped into that distinct feeling I had as a child when my father said, "Who said life was fair?" which left me feeling utterly alone and abandoned.

Once I realized and accepted that Myles was not going to be a part of my future, I was able to truly let go of my expectations.

The love and passion I had for this man, my newfound depth of emotion, my inexperience and emotional immaturity, all led me to believe we would be together despite our awkwardness. I didn't know I could feel this way about someone, especially without being in a relationship. Most everything occurred from a distance, through nonverbal communication. Neither of us possessed the skill to get past what was holding each of us back. He triggered me to the extreme, and it shut down any verbal communication between us, without which there was no hope of relating or properly expressing ourselves. On that last night I saw him, as the music he was playing rang out with the chorus, "He don't love you anymore," we both chose that moment to make eye contact, and I immediately knew that was exactly what he wanted to communicate to me. It felt like I had been kicked in the stomach. It was a shock that reverberated for the next six months. Before that night, I kept clinging to hope and chasing him, even though I would retreat with every awkward interaction, feeling rejected each time because of our lack of progress. I was caught in a loop until he broke the cycle.

He had finally let go, and it forced me to let go too, although not without catastrophic consequences for me. It unleashed the most prolonged traumatic response I've ever experienced: a six-month dissociative break from reality, during which time I took my life savings, both of my children's college funds, plus a ton of debt, and put it all in what turned out to be a bad "investment" (or in other words, a scam). It had, and will continue to have, severe financial repercussions that I will feel for many years. However, once I came out of denial about Myles, and about my whole life up to that point, I began to see that this was all about my learning, the learning I had never achieved as a child and young adult. My development had finally chugged back into action from a long period of dormancy.

The insights and realizations began to come very quickly (comparatively speaking, in a few years, instead of thirty), and I was able to understand what happened to me and what to do about it. It allowed me to focus on areas of my life that were, quite frankly, being neglected. Neglected! Ironically, his rejection of me had led me to come full circle. Instead of me feeling empty, it prefaced a sense of wholeness I have experienced only now, for the first time in my life, precisely because I had to learn to live without him. After grieving the loss and getting past the horrible, lingering sense of longing, I again noticed a shift in perspective and began to focus on other areas of my life that had been sidelined for some time, or that I had forgotten.

I missed being "in the zone" when creating something. I felt a sense of something almost blooming inside me. It was passion. It was not pursuit, which I had always felt before, like I was constantly chasing, in search of something (which of course was myself). I was no longer in the old habit of looking ahead to something, hoping I would attain some better future. This time I was excited about doing something just for me. It was a calling to do something greater than myself, to help others somehow, and also to present my ideas to the world in an artistic way, whereas before it was frightening for me to put myself out there for judgment.

Although I had been inspired before to do creative work, there seemed to be a purpose to what I was doing now, an unspecified purpose, such as just for the pleasure of doing it and pronouncing myself as a part of this world and participating in it, in a way I had never experienced before. I didn't feel like anyone had to validate me, as before, and neither did I need to prove myself to anyone. I felt inspired to do what I wanted, unrestrained. I felt content to be. It was a profound sense of peace. I had learned to truly let go. My learning from Myles was complete.

REFLECT ON LETTING GO

I invite you now to take out your journal and use it to reflect upon the changes (if any) in your life and how you feel about what you have learned so far. Pay special attention to whether you have noticed any "shifts" in your attitude, your outlook, your mindset or any changes you have noticed in your body and especially in your emotions. Take your newfound awareness and reflect on any changes you have made. Do you feel better? Have you changed any habits? Are you more mindful of your thoughts? Less triggered? Are those aches and pains subsiding? Are they getting worse? This can happen. I seemed to tense up right at the time that I was discharging emotional energy, before my body would begin to relax. At these times, I would also break out in rashes or hives—fun!

At least when the stress released and the emotional tension had finally dissipated, I would return to normal. A new normal, though. One that included tranquility and an inner sense of knowing and trusting myself. The shift is subtle yet simultaneously very impactful, because you have come to know yourself so intimately. Treat yourself with tenderness, caring and love because you need to be able to feel these things, especially about yourself, if you are to discover your purpose and passion.

9

Freedom: Where Do I Go from Here?

YOU WILL LIKELY revisit the steps from earlier chapters to find which are most effective for you as you progress in this work. Eventually, after you have felt some shifts in your consciousness, and the all-important release of emotion and tension in your body, you will get to the point that you can perhaps think, *What's next?* or, *Where do I go from here?* Once you are relieved of the effects of the trauma that held you back, what are you going to do with all of that freedom from repression, self-doubt and inhibition? Now you are truly free to choose the content of your life, but sometimes such a vast amount of freedom can paralyze you. It can be overwhelming to think about it. Discovering the potential for that freedom to be able to lead you to your purpose and passions is what this chapter is about.

Purpose and passion do not arise out of thin air. They are built on experiences, which is why I stress the importance of trying out the things that interest you. This mimics the early adult phase of life where one normally begins to pursue areas of interest. Purpose has the capacity for creating meaning in your life. Perhaps you will find something new that engages you and sustains your interest, providing that purpose as you move forward in your life. Alternatively, you may find a reignited interest in former passions, as I did. Start simple, and start somewhere.

Passion is something that you alone can determine. It is not important whether or not you have passions. You don't need a passion to live a fulfilling life, but it does add pleasure and satisfaction to it. Purpose is more value driven because it encompasses what is important to you. For instance, your job doesn't need to be your passion, but if you are doing something that is your purpose, it is more likely that you will feel fulfilled. Your career may not be your purpose, though. For some, it is raising a family, for others, volunteering or having hobbies, and for others, their relationships or perhaps even all of the above. As mentioned early on, giving yourself the time and space to investigate not only your trauma but also to explore your interests, abilities, aptitudes, passions and desires is key to building a rich life full of experience, perhaps even bliss, which feeds your soul. There are a couple of tools you can use to help you unlock that hidden desire or unbeknownst purpose.

DAYDREAMING

As I mentioned in previous chapters, I had a thriving fantasy life, and it was where most of my "living" was done as a child. I could do whatever or be whomever I wanted in my mind. It was the place where I could let go of all inhibitions, self-doubts and self-loathing, and ignore the inconveniences of reality. I dissociated this way almost on a daily basis. It was the most freedom I ever felt; however, I almost never dreamed of the future. Even as a teen, I had a hard time envisioning a future where I determined for myself what would happen. There was no point in thinking about it since someone would end up telling me what to do. This learned helplessness prevented me from having my own sense of control over my life.

The only daydream I remember having regarding my future was of me, dressed as a businesswoman in a red power suit, with a briefcase and heels, an up-do for my hair and glasses. This couldn't be further from the truth. I don't even wear glasses (*deadpans*). Seriously though, a Wall Street wunderkind I am not, as evidenced by my spectacular financial flop. I'm much more a sensitive artist, quite honestly. But what I realized my self-image did reflect was my tendency toward, and desire for, independence, autonomy and self-reliance, which my child mind interpreted as financial success and being seen as competent.

Sometimes these childhood dreams hold clues for us; other times they may just be fanciful. It's not a guarantee of what you want out of life, but it's another starting point, or another angle from which you can attend to your work, even if it's just by interpreting what the daydream from way back when represented. What did you want to be when you grew up? Did you ever picture yourself as an adult when you were a kid? Use your journal to write, or dictate into your phone, about any dreams and fantasies that you had, or things that you did in the past that you loved. How did you feel when thinking about it? Is it something you would want to try again?

My daydream informed me that my desire for independence and freedom were my most treasured values. It also told me about why setting aside money was always so important to me (for safety and security) because I never felt that I could rely on anyone else. Money was never a big motivator for me otherwise. I would also become filled with self-loathing whenever I failed at something, because I felt stupid and inferior, reminding me of my failure to attain independence. These old patterns reflected an outdated version of myself, but the daydream did help me figure out what was important to me.

By using the exercises in this book, you can work past these old patterns and peel away the layers of invisible trauma to reveal your true self. Your authentic self is who you are without the conditioning and the restraints that trauma from childhood neglect has placed upon you. In this state of being stripped down to your essential nature, you can decide what it is that you want. This is the beginning of the self-actualizing process, and revisiting your childhood fantasies can provide you some ideas or inspiration about where to start looking for your passion, and steer you toward fulfilling your dreams.

REDISCOVER WHAT MOST ENGAGED OR INSPIRED YOU

Returning to your childhood, this time to rediscover things that once fascinated you and activities or ideas that once engaged you, can help you in finding your passion. Revisiting those interests can help you remember the fun you had or the curiosity you felt when looking at something as simple as an ant carrying a leaf, or as sophisticated as appreciating a piece of music, art or the spellbinding absurdity of a Rube Goldberg machine. Allow yourself to reminisce, if you can, about the things that once excited you.

Remembering how you felt about something can help you feel these things again, reexperiencing your joys, or perhaps reigniting your passions. Pursuing your passions will align your mind, body, heart and soul to fulfill its calling. You will be putting your energies into something that raises your vibration, elevating you to a happier, healthier life, because all of your efforts are being put toward life-affirming activities, creating "good vibes" at all levels, which in turn creates greater life satisfaction. These elements all go hand-in-hand. Having nurturing, fulfilling relationships and a job that engages you, whether it's the people or the actual work you love, and engaging in hobbies, activities or volunteerism creates the uplift that elevates your life to the point of self-actualization.

WHAT IS IT THAT YOU MOST WANT?

Ask yourself, what is it that you want out of your relationships, your occupation, your creative aspirations, your active outlets, your sexual desires and any other important areas of your life? What are, or were, your dreams? How can you achieve these things? Use your journal to record your thoughts. Then, begin to plan. What is required? Looking for a new job? Pursuing an education? Contemplating the logistics and contingencies of going backpacking around the world? Setting aside time to plan the next steps for something like preparing applications? Active and mutual communication with your partner or family to cooperatively set aside time for these things?

Can you carve out time for yourself to actually contemplate, produce or compose a creative work or new project? This is not limited to the arts; science and technology can offer creative opportunities as well. Can you find an expressive outlet, whether it's singing in the shower or in the car on the way to work, or actually joining a band or recording music yourself? Can you spare thirty minutes to devote entirely to your children, to play and connect with them without any other distractions or commitments interfering? Or how about the same for yourself, taking thirty minutes, say, right after work, to relax, decompress or do something you enjoy in order to reconnect to yourself?

Take time to plan how you can fit these new behaviors into your busy schedule, to make them habits. How can you find the time or create the energy to be able to take on more and therefore feel like you are getting more out of your life without feeling exhausted or defeated before you begin? Building on habits you already have, such as an exercise regimen, is a good place to start. Can you fit in anything else during that time, or dedicate time to other important things as well? See the above example of singing in the shower or the car, or maybe even on the treadmill if you have a home gym. Perhaps you can switch up your workout occasionally by watching some YouTube videos to learn K-pop dancing, or go shoot some hoops with friends. Try sharing childcare by rotating with other parents on weekends sometimes to get in some "me" time. Think of how else you might be able to help yourself. Try to enlist the help of the people in your life, and in turn you may be able to reciprocate to help them to get more out of their lives too.

If you align your energies, this all becomes possible. When you are working with—rather than against—yourself, energy flows naturally. If something doesn't align with you, or you find yourself feeling inner resistance to something, don't do it! Find something else to do, or find some other way to achieve what you want. Rearrange your schedule. Think early morning study, late evening practice or exercise on your lunch break, for example. As I mentioned before, start somewhere. Pick one thing and begin, so you don't get overwhelmed before you even start. Take small steps, tackling one thing at a time, and simplify your life. Take a walk in the morning before work to set an intention for the day. Another idea is to have a simple, daily, easily achievable goal, so that once you have done it, you are already winning, everyday! The uplift from that can help you plan to set aside specific times to work toward accomplishing your bigger projects.

CLEARING OUT THE JUNK

Clearing and managing your schedule can help with planning ahead, but getting rid of "stuff" (especially kid's toys, I find) is also a good way to progress with your goals. Clear the clutter from your mind— and your environment—to get results from the changes in your life. You are changing your life from the inside out. It starts internally, but eventually you can see the positive changes you've made reflected in your external circumstances as well, by clearing out junk and making physical space, which can allow for more internal "space" because you will not feel so overwhelmed. Take things one step at a time.

RETURN TO PLAY

Once you clear all the internal "gunk" as well as the external "junk," you will have prepared yourself for more play. Play is not only what can spark inspiration; a lot of learning also happens during play. Play energizes you, and when the so-called "happy accidents" occur, you internalize that positive energy. What did you like to play with when you were a kid? Can you return to that activity, or is there an equivalent in adulthood that you can do instead? Play can happen in an adult context as well if you consider things like art, music and sports.

Play is a mixture of fun, engagement and learning. Play in adulthood reconnects us to our former interests but also, perhaps more importantly, to our past and our true selves. It allows us time to relax, recharge and to not worry about the outcome, while also learning, rejuvenating and possibly even entering a state of "flow," where you lose track of time while you focus exclusively on an engaging task, hobby or activity, often one that you love. Make time for more play! Play is a gateway to passion and to making your dreams come true, by letting go of expectations, surrendering to the process or perhaps even the game, and making room for the visitation of inspiration.

SURRENDER

Surrendering to the process combines the concepts of trust, letting go and acceptance. I think of it as allowing your soul to breathe. Trusting yourself gives you the courage to continue this journey, which allows you to trust the universe to provide for you and the faith that life will work out. Letting go of expectations is also necessary and is more of a mental process, but letting go of the physical manifestation of angst, trapped in the body, is just as important. Acceptance of how all the things that came before now have unfolded in your life is also essential in order to have hope for your future. The integration of these elements culminates in surrender.

Surrendering will provide the greatest payoff in terms of seeking an outcome, although I would caution against having a specific outcome in mind. Actively searching for happiness is a recipe for not finding happiness. Happiness or, more accurately, contentment, especially with oneself, is a natural result of focusing on your own development. It is a state of being, not a state of mind or simply a heart-centered feeling. Feelings are fleeting, although negative ones can be persistent when not integrated. Happiness, however, encompasses the whole of your being. It is a state that creates an energetic vibration stemming from a sense of peace, self-acceptance and detachment from forces outside of your control.

At first, I thought surrender was easy. I embraced the process because I wanted to hurry it along in order not to lose my chance with Myles, because I could see the writing on the wall. It didn't work, at least not in time, and the real surrendering had to happen after it all fell apart. Saying goodbye to Myles was simultaneously a process in grieving, a mind-bending flight into dissociative fantasy and a coming-to-terms with growth and what it means to be alive. What it unlocked in me was surrender. I needed to be cracked open and broken down to my barest essence, breaking away all the (perceived) societal expectations and familial conditioning, in order to repair myself.

It was truly ego-death. It was a realization that my life was a façade communally built by my parents, my family, my friends, society and me! The sheer magnitude of this realization was impossible to bear, and it pulverized my psyche. I was forced to surrender by getting to a breaking point, in order to open myself up to a life of freedom and meaning. However, it doesn't need to be something this *dramatic* (last time, I pinky-swear) to be effective in changing your life. Although it was personally and financially catastrophic, unspeakably painful, and a shocking recognition of denial, it was also life-altering and granted me the ultimate freedom: freedom from fear. I could finally decompress from the decades of built-up tension, doubt and fear that ruled my life and wake up to a new realization that my life could be different. I was never before able to conceptualize the broader scope of experience that was possible and available to me.

Surrendering to the process is sometimes easier said than done. Creating your new life requires your persistence, patience, perseverance, practice (there's that word again) and perhaps a touch of humility. How do you expect to be good at something without practice? You can use mindfulness (staying in the present moment) as well as gratitude (counting your blessings) and affirmations about your life as it stands right now, to remind yourself of all that you have and all of the progress you have made. Those of us who somehow interpreted events very differently in childhood than was intended by our parents, or inherited beliefs that were very strong, be they our own, our parents', our community's or our society's "rules," or we just never felt like we were "enough" for various reasons, unfortunately (or, perhaps, fortunately) have to do the detective work to discover who we really are and what life really is.

Life doesn't have to be what others, or perhaps even you, say it is or expect it to be. Your life is of your own making, created moment by moment, and taking responsibility for that means that you get to change your life in whatever way serves you and those you love best, which will benefit all of you in the long run. You'll be better prepared even when things don't go your way. I make it sound simple, but of course that does not mean it will be easy. It can be *easier*, however, if you are not fighting yourself, first and foremost, and secondarily if you are not fighting your family, friends and so on.

So, set yourself up for success. Accepting your unique challenges, such as the amount of time you have to devote to this, the cooperation (or lack thereof) of others in your life and your willingness to attend to your practices, will go a long way in taking off any pressure to meet a real or even an imagined timeline. Deal with one issue at a time as it arises. Remind yourself as well as others of the importance of what you are doing, not to mention the benefits. Accepting also that there may be an unpleasant impact from the memories being brought up or emotions you may experience in the process will help move you through this journey faster than fighting it. Remember that once these feelings are recognized, felt and let go, they become integrated and they no longer have a hold over you. The emotional impact is neutralized and they simply become learning experiences.

Some things that can help are to remember to have gratitude for the abundance in your life and to realize that the power lies with you to find wholeness within yourself, experience the happiness borne from contentment and to wield your personal power. Try going in with a mindset of discovery rather than expectation, by seeing challenges as learning opportunities and knowing that your work will effect positive changes in your life, which will be unique for each person and may look different than what you might have anticipated. Take heart in the fact that you have the courage to take this path. Trust and surrender to what the universe has in store for you. That's what this whole journey has been about, anyway: discovering your trauma, discovering yourself, truly discovering life. Therein lies the path to discovering your passion.

PASSION VS. PURPOSE

Living with passion sounds blissful and effortless, but the truth is, you must complete your personal work in order to unlock your passions. They are tied to purpose, but purpose and passions are not the same thing. Passion is driven by desire. Purpose fuels your life and gives it direction, but it is not determined by what you do. It is determined by who you are and what you want. However, your worth is not contingent on what you "do with your life." Your existence is not defined by anything or anyone. Your worth is intrinsic and inherent. Once you realize this, you will find that what personally drives you, piques your interest or even something that just happened to lie in your path one day unexpectedly, can become your life's work (like writing a book, *wink*). You begin to notice that the things that resonate with you most begin to show up for you more often, and you begin to notice this feeling of *alignment*.

These experiences are called synchronicities, and they happen more and more as you align yourself with what feels right for you and how you want to live. Suddenly, things take less effort. You know what it's like to be "in the zone" or "in flow" as you have heard others describe. When you work at something important to you, you feel more energized and motivated to do more and continue doing it. And boom! Suddenly you discover purpose where you weren't even looking for it.

Purpose is something that engages you and gives you the motivation to continue a pursuit, just to seek the results of your efforts. Sometimes it transforms into, or leads to, a passion, sometimes not. Writing this book and serving others in the capacity of a counselor, for example, is my purpose, but it is not my passion. It engages me and motivates me, but what really lights a fire inside me is music, dance, art and filmmaking. Those are my passions, and I can do these things as a hobby, just for the joy of exploring, and with no particular outcomes expected. Also, my hobbies can be combined with my purpose in the context of workshops, where artistic expression is the focus.

It was trying different things and deciding what was truly important to me that made me able to discern the difference between passion and purpose and to pursue them for different reasons. Passions are what I love doing anytime throughout life. Purpose is often more practical, in that it is something you have discovered that engages you, makes use of your skills and sustains your attention or interest. I know an insurance salesman, whose purpose was derived from comprehensively learning his business and doing very well for himself so that he could have the lifestyle he wanted for his family, his true passion. Like many, he pursued a career in something that he could engage in so that he could spend his time outside of that, enjoying what he truly loved.

For some, however, pursuing passions can lead you to your purpose. For me, it was by taking charge of my life, and responsibility for my future career and happiness, that I rediscovered my passions of music and dance. Once I became separated from my husband, I wasted no time before going out to clubs to dance. I began to embrace other forms of dance as well, with ecstatic dance being of particular help in releasing emotion and allowing unabashed expression that had previously been stifled. It is this long-lost expression that came to the surface and began making a home in my heart and head. I received more ideas and inspiration than I had had in many years. An idea for a book began to percolate in my mind. I didn't have any writing background, training or experience, but shortly thereafter, an invitation for a free book-writing challenge showed up on my Facebook feed. I'm sure you get where this is going. Oddly enough, it was pursuing my passion that led indirectly to writing these words, my newfound purpose, because an opening up had occurred inside me that allowed me to expand my horizons and to believe that something else was possible for me.

I had rediscovered passions that I had not even realized were my own because I never indulged them. I have always loved music and dance but had compartmentalized them into parts of my life where it was "appropriate," such as at parties or listening on my way to and from work. The simple fact was that the relaxation and true joy of getting lost in a project were missing from my life and experienced at only a few times, which I treasured. I didn't give myself permission to allow that kind of time to be spent on my own passions and would only indulge in activities that were perceived by me to be implicitly or explicitly "approved" by my husband, or when it met some goal (such as making a wedding gift for my best friend). This is not how I live my life anymore, and I hope this illustrates the self-imposed prison that I created for myself, and that I needed to escape in order to "find myself," or just love myself, really. I needed to allow myself to develop and let my own energy, intuition and inspiration guide me toward self-actualization.

Engage and Inspire Exercise

I want you to consider what it is that engages you and inspires you. Perhaps one thing does both, but consider whether there is anything that you can do to make use of your skills that aligns with your interests or taps into your personal experiences in a way that you can pass on to others. On a piece of paper or in your journal, draw two columns. Title one "Engages" and the other "Inspires." This illustrates the difference between what has the potential to be your purpose and what is most definitely your passion. You can decide whether either is worth pursuing or just participating in. You never know where it can lead you. I went back to school, not once but twice, in order to seek purpose in what I was doing. The thing is, if I hadn't gone the first time and decided it wasn't for me, I likely would never have conceived of going down the path of counseling psychology because the first path led me to the second. When one door closes, another opens.

If you have self-limiting beliefs like I had, due to unresolved trauma and conditioning from family and society, it is very liberating to finally be taking life into your own hands and steering the ship. After all, finding your passion is about finding what lights you up. But something inexplicable seems to start happening as well. Doors begin to open that you didn't see before, partly because a shift has taken place from your previous perspective that didn't allow you to perceive an opportunity that may have been in front of you, either because you didn't notice it or you didn't believe it was possible to pursue it. I finally committed to studying psychology after rejecting my first course of study, but initially I had not considered it possible.

Something else is at play as well. Suddenly, but slowly, new things start to pop up one by one—whether they are job opportunities, new ideas, chances to participate in the arts or sports, or some community event—that show up at just the right time for you to take advantage of them, or things line up so that what you end up doing is the right choice, even though you may initially have felt unsure about your trajectory. Self-doubt is pretty much guaranteed at some point in this process. However, by trying things, you narrow the search by dismissing some things and accepting others, so that you eventually learn to trust your intuition and *know* when something is the right thing to do. And that's where life gets really interesting.

This definitely doesn't all happen at once, and it's not that your every desire is fulfilled and every wish is granted. You're simply better able to sense, understand and feel that perceptual shift in yourself, and it often shows up in your life as previously unforeseen opportunities arising and sometimes noticing coincidences or synchronicities that are borderline mystical in their nature and timing. This intuition is an inner knowing, an instinct if you will, that you learn to trust unquestioningly. I have manifested far too many things—some big, some small—in recent years to not have noticed it as an ongoing phenomenon in my life. It is conceiving of something desirable and then letting that feeling, that idea or that intention go, with no expectation of it appearing, yet maintaining positivity and a belief in its possibility. This is where the magic happens, and it seems to work in concert with your better or newfound ability to feel, understand and perceive things with the belief that you can have what you want in your life by doing what you feel is right.

Becoming *attuned* to yourself and the energies that govern life really can give you incredible personal power by altering your energy. You know those "vibes" that I mentioned? That is all energy, and you have control over how yours is emitted, by maintaining your positivity or neutrality and managing your negativity. I have guided you to use the strategies in this book to help you wield the power and energy that you possess. It is all within the realm of possibility to achieve awareness of yourself, and to find wholeness, happiness and personal power. It is a matter of choice that lies solely with you. You can choose to grow, to live up to your potential, to raise your vibration, to transform yourself, to self-actualize and to focus your energy on the things that inspire you. Most importantly, you can choose to foster and nurture healthy relationships, and spread love to others in a way that reaches further than you imagined possible and fulfills your destiny of conquering fear through the triumph of love.

CONCLUSION

It takes courage to make changes in your life. I'll tell you, though, that despite all of the stress, uncertainty, doubt, pain and suffering, the effort was still worth it for me. Spending your life hiding from yourself is no way to live. Doing the work is preferable to standing still, and it takes patience, because the process can sometimes be arduous and take longer than you might expect or hope. At times, it felt like contraction and expansion, or like the pain, grief and despair was coming in waves. Each time, however, I noticed that the severity of these episodes decreased incrementally. I experienced regression, too, returning to an earlier phase, or falling back on old habits of thinking, acting and feeling. I simply kept up the work.

I hope this book encourages you to keep up the work too. You will likely cycle through the steps similarly to how I did; however, you may do it in a different order or place more emphasis on certain chapters, exercises or activities. Do whatever works best for you. It can be hard, it can be challenging and it takes courage, but if I can do it, so can you. Use the ideas in this book to your advantage, by doing the tasks that spur you to action or even by tackling the easiest things first to build some confidence and momentum. Whether you use only one idea in this book or all of them, just keep doing it. Make it a habit. Practice, practice, practice. This is the way to get through your self-directed therapy more quickly to finally move past your trauma.

Becoming aware and building resilience are the first steps. You can start like I did, by making connections between my memories and my present emotional state, and then use the ACEs study to determine how trauma, due to emotional neglect or any other trauma you may have experienced, has affected you. Learning to actually feel the emotion and sit with it, just letting it happen, is definitely a difficult task but necessary for you to move past your trauma. You can use grounding and breathing exercises to help you through this. Getting to the other side of that emotion, by working through it, takes the emotional charge away from it and frees you from fear.

The next step is accepting your life circumstances as they are right now. You can challenge your perspective by noticing how you talk to yourself, and how you view your life circumstances. You can think about how perspective forms your view of life. Being able to see from another's perspective is a valuable skill and a building block for empathy. Empathy is valuable because if you can feel something of what someone else feels, then you can relate to them, hence you are better able to build relationships and foster intimacy. Forgiving others for their faults—as well as yourself—helps give power and agency back to you. Reframing your experiences—from seeing yourself as a victim to having gratitude for all the people and things that enrich your life—creates a powerful shift that promotes connectedness to self, which in turn allows you to connect with others.

You can then dive in deeper and begin the inner-child work of learning to self-soothe and regulate your emotions. The practice of reparenting is also vital in order to learn to be your own emotional support. Then you can move onto embodiment practices. Anything from typical weight-bearing exercises and cardiovascular activities or sports to martial arts, hiking, yoga and dance can work. Creative or expressive arts like music, art and drama can also be used as therapy, particularly in more specific, intense and focused forms, if mindfully and intentionally used to express emotions that have long been repressed. Music actually took me by surprise, with songs appearing in my dreams. I had deprived myself of a creative outlet for so long, thinking that I couldn't fit it into my life, that my brain decided to find another conduit for me on its own. This helped me realize what I was missing, and I began to reevaluate my life and what was important to me. You can begin trying new things, or going back to activities that you once enjoyed.

The truth is that all of these concepts can be summed up as taking responsibility for your life, which could also be described as a reality check or, even more simply, as growing up. Once you do this, it gives you the confidence that you can create a new life for yourself. To better understand what it is that you want, and to hope for a better future, you must have a firm idea of your identity. Your identity will inform you of your values, which can in turn provide you some direction. You can therefore have hope for a new life driven by who you are and what is important to you.

Using body-based (somatic) healing, you can promote mind-body connection by focusing on the expressive arts mentioned above, plus things like breathwork and vocal work. It is also important to consider other areas of care that may help you, such as traditional Western medicine, physical therapies, psychology and naturopathy, or more esoteric practices like acupuncture, iridology and reflexology. The list goes on. I encourage you to continue whatever therapies work for you. Seeing a doctor, counselor or therapist is a great idea, but remember to continue some or all of the exercises outlined in this book on your own as well, because all of these treatments work better together, as each of them has the potential to reveal unknown information to you. Holistic care treats the body as a whole, and consideration of your physical, mental and emotional well-being is paramount. Being a whole person is the necessary ingredient for healthy relationships, based on an authentic connection between people, because you have a connection to yourself and to your own needs.

In reflecting on your journey, you can focus on your present circumstances to keep yourself grounded and remind yourself of why you took on this challenge. Focusing on the present moment is valuable because you don't waste your time worrying about the future or fretting about the past, while accepting the circumstances of your life without judgment. You can learn to trust yourself in this process of self-discovery, and in so doing make it possible for you to trust others in a healthy way. Letting go of expectations builds on trust, because it is required in order to believe that everything will work out.

Using daydreams and surrendering to the process, which is a combination of accepting all life experiences and trusting that they are serving your greater good, while letting go of an expected outcome, can instill a sense of peace. Identifying your purpose and passion will guide you toward living your dreams and is the final phase of the journey. You can allow yourself to be inspired or intrigued by something, guided by your own inner knowledge of what you want and what is important to you, and follow that calling to do something that your soul is calling for or, at least, that which draws your attention and keeps you engaged. You can then earn a living in a consciously chosen field and focus on your passions outside of work, if necessary.

You can start this process now, but it starts by healing yourself, and in order to do that you need to be able to take care of number one first. It is ironic for someone like me, who hid my despair and depression behind a (figurative, pre-COVID) "mask," that I am rather fond of the analogy of using the airplane emergency procedure of putting the oxygen mask on yourself first, and only then tending to your loved ones, as being good advice for life. The wisdom of the analogy is that you can't help others until you have helped yourself. Only when you have healed yourself can you truly take care of others, especially children, who learn from your example. It means taking responsibility for acknowledging what happened to you and how you responded to it, and then taking on the work to repair the damage. Only you can be responsible for your own thoughts, feelings and behaviors, no matter what happened to you. It is imperative to take that responsibility in order for your sense of self to develop and for your healing and your growth to take place.

Taking responsibility for yourself is the crux of taking back your power, or perhaps even claiming it for the first time. Recognizing, appreciating and loving yourself is a requirement for happiness. The other connections in life, such as relationships, family and friends, are what add to your happiness and fill your life with experiences from which to learn and grow. Despite all the pain and suffering, I wouldn't trade my experience for any other now. Experience has been my school, while family, friends, lost loves, even acquaintances and especially my children have been my best teachers. I have an appreciation for all that I have and all that has been shared with me. I am proud of the work I have done. You, too, can be proud of whatever work you choose to take on, which can have deeply meaningful and positive impacts for yourself, your family and others in your circle.

Tracing, identifying and taking responsibility for your emotions are what guide you on the path to overcoming your trauma. Once you have achieved wholeness, happiness and personal power, the world opens up to you in ways you may have never experienced. People treat you differently once they see you as the best version of yourself, who is fully participating in life. I have had more people approach me to socialize than ever before in my life, and I think it is partly because of me holding my head up high now with my shoulders back instead of doing my best to disappear into the background. I'm also sure it is partly because of the energy I now possess, which undoubtedly influences my posture and conveys an aura of confidence.

Instead of hiding behind behaviors that mask your fears, anger and anxiety, or being overwhelmed by the immense suffering and despair of depression, you are unafraid to speak your mind, stand up for yourself and pursue your dreams without undue compromise. You present your best self to people without subjugating yourself to their desires and demands. You learn to set boundaries, trust others and trust yourself. Essentially, you grow. You grow in your capacity to love and to give. You become able to form and experience happy, healthy relationships. You are able to be at peace.

This is what I want for anyone taking this path. The tools and exercises in this book helped me achieve this. Developing self-awareness and self-love leads to a more meaningful experience, a peaceful existence and a fulfilling life. My whole motivation behind writing this book is to help people who, like me, experienced emotional neglect as a child and suffered its pervasive consequences in their lives. It is for those who have walked a similar path to mine and want some guidance on how best to navigate it. You have taken the first step in your journey home to yourself. You should be proud of your courage for taking on this most important work. Be gentle with yourself. Use the support network you have in your life to set aside time for yourself to investigate and explore your past, yourself and your relationships in order to attain your goals. There is no greater cause than healing yourself, so that you can connect and relate with others, or perhaps even serve others.

I can continue to serve you as well. If you need support through the process of healing from your trauma, I offer services as a counselor. I especially like to encourage the use of expressive arts, music and dance to help unlock and express the repressed emotion trapped in the body. For more information, you can go to my website at traumatotriumph.ca. If you have your support system in place and are ready to take on this work on your own, I say all the power to you, because you already have it within you to do it. I would be delighted to know how your journey progresses. Please don't hesitate to contact me via my website to tell me all about it. I would love to hear from you. I wish you bon voyage on your unique life journey!

Made in the USA
Monee, IL
18 February 2023

27491886R00095